The Cure
of Childhood
Leukemia

The
Cure
of
Childhood
Leukemia

Into the Age
of Miracles

John Laszlo, M.D.

National Vice President for Research
American Cancer Society

Rutgers University Press
New Brunswick, New Jersey

Library of Congress Cataloging-in-Publication Data

Laszlo, John, 1931–
    The cure of childhood leukemia : into the age of miracles / John
Laszlo.
        p.   cm.
    Includes bibliographical references and index.
    ISBN 0-8135-2186-6
    1. Leukemia in children—Research—History.   2. Leukemia in
children—Treatment—History.   I. Title.
RJ416.L4L38   1995
618.92'9941906—dc20   94-47285
                                                                                    CIP

British Cataloging-in-Publication information available

Dedicated to the thousands of families and the hundreds of scientists who were united by a common goal—to eliminate leukemia as a dread disease

Contents

Contents

Preface

The cure for childhood leukemia is a singular event in the history of medicine. Singular because it proves that cancer *can* be cured, a significant achievement that opens the way to victory over the many other faces of the disease. Singular too because of the way the cure emerged. In our society, it is often only the final result, the bottom line, that captures attention. So let it be told that, with childhood leukemia, there was no such thing as *the discovery* of a cure—rather there was the brilliant assembly of a series of small, endlessly persevering steps forward that led to success. This book is about how it happened, who did it, and why they kept on trying.

The history of the cure of childhood leukemia is so recent that we do not need to reconstruct or extrapolate from scattered records. Most of the physicians and scientists who did the major work are still alive. So are many of their patients—the best testimonial to the success of the endeavor. Their recollections serve as the chief, rich source for telling this story.

I will, of course, draw on many hundreds of published papers in the medical literature, but these papers (as any researcher will tell you) provide only the formal side of what happened. They do not explain all the reasoning behind the experiments or the motives of the researchers. The papers do not tell us how the author got the nugget of the idea from a hallway conversation with someone in a different field or from a technician who did the experiment the wrong way. The papers cannot show the connections between leukemia research and work on other cancers or to biomedical research in general. Yet, to tell the story properly, we must take account of those interrelationships: biomedical research is a whole, not just a collection of separate investigations into different disease entities. Biomedical discoveries do not come with labels on them—this one for diabetes, this one for transplants, this one for AIDS, this one for leukemia. There is a process of thinking and doing—from hunches and astute observations, to basic research ideas, to constructing and executing definitive and ethical experiments, to carefully analyzing and interpreting the data, and finally to finding the right applications. There are no shortcuts. This is especially true when it comes to human experimentation, in which the participants have their own individual characteristics, including their personal willingness and motivation for entering into a research program.

For all that we like to think of scientific discovery as the fruit of the dispassionate search for truth, the fact is that science is a passionate business. The passion for knowledge and for results can cut both ways. It can lead to wishful thinking, to misreading and warping of research, even on rare occasions to outright fraud and deceit—that is why scientists have created elaborate systems of peer review and publication to check and recheck one another's work. Much more often, though, it is a constructive and energetic passion that leads researchers to spend weekends and evenings in the laboratory or hospital, harnessing intellect and emotion together. We shall see this powerful drive for knowledge and tangible results revealed in the lives and words of the scientists who did the work that brought victory over childhood leukemia.

Scientists often compare the pleasures of their work to the satisfaction of filling in a jigsaw puzzle. The puzzle posed by leukemia is far from finished. But we do have the outline, and the shape and form of the picture are becoming clear enough to give us confidence that we are nearer the end than the beginning. Good as the jigsaw puzzle metaphor is, however, it fails to convey just how messy the reality is. The leukemia puzzle is an enormously complex, perverse one, where pieces are missing, overlap, cancel each other out, have blurry edges, even come from different boxes! Filling in just a small corner of the puzzle demands doggedness, imagination, and an open mind. For example, how could a quirk of medical geography—the peculiarly high rate of an unusual form of leukemia (T-cell) found in southern Japan *and* in the Caribbean—have anything to do with epidemics of leukemia in chickens? Yet the pieces were indeed linked. In both the rare human leukemia and the common poultry disease, a virus could be pinpointed as the reason why normal blood cells became leukemic. That recognition of virally triggered leukemias in turn made it possible to develop a vaccine that now routinely protects pet cats from yet another deadly form of the disease, feline leukemia.

The completion of that patch of the leukemia puzzle is, thus far, irrelevant to most human leukemias—their cause remains a mystery. But that little segment teaches some valuable lessons. Successful research may draw on the wits and skills of scientists in a dozen disciplines. It swings back and forth among studies on groups of people, individual patients, animals, cells, tiny parts of cells, chemicals, and viruses. We can never be sure where the next major advance will come from, where one line of work will hook up with another. We can only marvel at the richness, diversity, power, and universality of science and have hope that—as it has in the past—it will lead to the understanding and cure of disease.

The physical laws of nature are often wondrously simple once they are unraveled. By contrast, the achievement of medical cures seems more complex and asymmetric. The end result is important, to be sure, but that seems somehow both more and less than the sum of the parts. More because it is the outcome, the saving of lives, that is the real triumph; less because, in retrospect, the result seems to have been found more than once, by more than one person or group. While there is enough satisfaction and reward to go around, in my view there is insufficient recognition of the greatness of individual achievement, particularly when medical research requires close cooperation among many talented people.

My goal in this book is not to establish historical priority of discovery for this person or another. That would—if it is possible at all—require a very long and technical study. Rather, I want to explore the roles of some of the individual scientists, these ordinary yet extraordinary people who became part of a great medical success story. What does it take to achieve that greatness? When is it recognized? Most of these researchers came out of families with no tradition of scientific involvement. Each had to make his or her own way. Each had separate inspirations. Yet all were willing to gamble at early stages in their careers; all were incredible optimists—to the point of foolishness, some said. To see the battle from the field as they saw it permits us to share their joys and their sorrows, and perhaps to dream of what we ourselves can do in other campaigns that lie ahead.

I want to examine some of the redundancies and blind alleys as well as the significant insights and events, to show how the tangled strands of scientific discovery come together in practice, how one finding catalyzes others, often in rapid succession. The story is a complex one; as I move from one individual or group's story to another, it may seem that I am backtracking or leaving loose ends. But that's exactly how the researchers themselves felt, and it would be misleading to tidy up what happened.

Every time I contemplate this story, I am astonished by it. At the beginning, less than a lifetime ago, *every* child and adult with leukemia was doomed. *Today, we can cure most of the children.* If we knew then what we know now, we could have saved so many of those beautiful children. If we knew now what we shall surely discover soon, how many more people could be saved? But the success of the work on childhood leukemia goes much further, for the principles first learned there are being applied to other forms of cancer and saving still more lives. Leukemia research has been the stalking horse for effective treatments of Hodgkin's disease, lymphomas (cancers of the lymph glands), and other common kinds of cancers. Standing now on the threshold of a new era, we can honestly hope that, early in the next millennium, leukemia will become curable not only in children but in all who are afflicted with this terrible disease. Truly we have moved into the age of miracles.

I am grateful to my assistants Deborah Siebels and Mary Ellen Banisch for their skillful help with the drafts of the manuscript; to Ian Ballantine, who had confidence in the book; Betty Ballantine and Karen Reeds, who helped immensely with its organization and clarity; and to Judith Weber for her help and encouragement. The Rockefeller Foundation in Bellagio provided a brief haven from other distractions. The American Cancer Society gave me the freedom to write the book: the Society is not responsible for its content but will receive its proceeds.

Because the information in this book is primarily from personal knowledge and interviews, special thanks go to each of the principals. They shared with me their personal lives—we had long been professional colleagues and friends. They had the opportunity to review their own chapters and to correct my errors or indiscretions. A selected bibliography is available at the back of the book to amplify specific topics. I hope that the many other scientists who have contributed extensively to this field will understand that a single book for a general audience cannot do justice to all who deserve recognition. In particular, the role of large medical cooperative groups in studying large numbers of children has been greatly condensed in this account. Thanks go also to St. Jude Children's Research Hospital for providing assistance in reaching several of their successful "alumni," who provided their own stories as early leukemia survivors, and to several of the other lucky ones who did the same. In some instances the names of patients have been changed. The unknown soldiers and heroes in this war are the members of the American public, who support leukemia and other cancer research via their taxes and their personal donations to agencies such as the American Cancer Society and the Leukemia Society.

Prologue

At that moment—now almost forty years ago—it was impossible to tell whether Samuel Beard regarded me as an ally or an adversary. He had just explained to me that he had led a full and satisfying life, although he seemed to wonder whether the difference in our ages kept me from understanding what that meant to him. What he was absolutely clear about was that he had no wish to endure further discomfort—either from his leukemia or from any more treatment. The new chemotherapy we had designed to destroy his leukemic cells was only making him more miserable.

Two plastic intravenous tubes were feeding fresh whole blood into the veins of both arms, while a suction tube coming out of his nose extracted (both his own and other people's) blood from his bleeding stomach. The firm rubber nasal tube resembled a convoluted red proboscis as it curved out from one nostril over his upper lip, across his cheekbones, and over his ear. Sam could not avoid tugging at this intruder, yet it caused him sharp pain each time. He coughed up more dark blood around the nasal tube, which passed by the back of his throat. He excreted still more in frequent bloody stools and in his urine. Red, purple, and green blotches from spontaneous bruising covered his skin. His own blood lacked sufficient platelets to keep him from bleeding—hence the need for fresh blood transfusions. Blood was coming out as fast as we could pour it in. In short sentences he pleaded with me; he wanted to leave this world as soon as possible.

What were my choices? After all, he lacked normal white blood cells to fight infections, lacked the tiny blood platelets that plug blood vessels and prevent bleeding, and the red blood cells he had were all courtesy of blood transfusion. All of this was typical of normal bone marrow that had been ousted by leukemic cells. I could stop giving blood and antibiotics as he begged, and then he would probably be dead from loss of blood or infection in a day or two. He could be reminded that he had come to our Leukemia Service at the National Cancer Institute on his own volition, specifically to receive the latest experimental treatment in hopes of prolonging his life; that was what we were doing and would continue to do until the end if he remained willing. I did explain that the new treatments might still work, but it was too early to tell and that perhaps another week of tough sledding would be needed before the normal cells in his own bone marrow would have an opportunity to recover from the effects of chemotherapy. He decided to endure, but let me know that it was against his "better judgment." I did not know whether any other patient so sick with leukemia had ever improved, but I didn't need to spell that out for him. He needed to hope and we were all hoping that each new day would be better than the last.

We spent a lot of time together during the next seven to ten days and nights, agonizing in our separate ways. Even the experienced nurses on the leukemia ward were unable to draw blood out of his ravaged arm veins for laboratory tests, which forced me to draw the most essential blood samples from veins in the groin, ankles, and neck, leaving ugly marks. Finger sticks were used to get precious drops of blood for daily blood counts. Bone marrow samples had to be obtained periodically. This was done under sterile conditions by cleansing the skin with a rotary motion using an antiseptic gauze sponge, numbing the area with a local anesthetic, and pushing a large hollow needle into his breastbone or pelvis and suctioning out marrow cells into a syringe. He dreaded going through each such procedure, as the suctioning was sharply painful and the procedure invariably left a bruise. Repeated bruises on his hips made it uncomfortable to lie on one side or the other.

Sam's family members required at least an equal amount of my time. They too were divided about the wisdom of vigorously seeking the rare remission. Few gamblers would wager their money on such long odds. Furthermore, I had to admit that, if a remission could be achieved, it might last only weeks or a few months, during which Sam might be fully well, but then slip right back into the same dreadful situation. The family struggled to find the "right" thing to do when, in fact, the only thing they could do was to be there, to support him with their loving presence. This they did very well and very naturally. They often needed reassurance that they were doing the best that they could for Sam. "Just be yourself" was the best advice I could offer.

Sam persevered, and so did his family and his doctors and nurses. We gave him more than thirty units (pints) of fresh blood from family, friends, and unknown blood donors, completely refilling his "tank" of blood three times in that week. He bled from the bowel. He bled into the retina of both eyes, obscuring his vision. His mouth, tongue, and throat were raw and sore; it was very painful even to swallow his own saliva. We fed him with liquid formula nourishments through the ubiquitous stomach tube.

Then the laboratory called one afternoon to see if we could send another blood sample so they could check it again, because there might have been a mix-up of tubes. The counts appeared to have improved so remarkably that the technicians believed there must have been a laboratory error. By pricking the side of one of Sam's bruised fingers with a needle, I managed to draw a few drops of blood into capillary glass tubes, sufficient to repeat the counts and to look at the cells under the microscope. Where Sam previously had only large and very wild-looking leukemic cells in place of his normal white blood cells, now the leukemia cells had totally disappeared! And normal white blood cells and platelets were now in evidence. There was much to celebrate, but we were too tired to manage more than smiles of relief and gratitude.

Within a day or two Sam could smile too, because I removed the tube from his nose that had bothered him day and night. In his own mind, the tube had come to be more important than even life or death. Dried blood had crusted in his nostril, and I inadvertently hurt him in pulling out the tube. I remembered my own discomfort at having my laboratory partner in medical school insert and remove a stomach tube when we were learning to do such procedures on each other. We suffered through the gagging, choking, nasal irritation, watery eyes—and we were healthy young people. Sam was greatly relieved when it was done. He might have given all his worldly possessions to be thus freed. We released his arms, which had been secured with adhesive tape to bulky padded arm boards to protect the intravenous tubes that had been his lifeline. Now happiness came simply in flexing his fingers, slowly bending his arms, and scratching his face.

Sam left the hospital within a week. When I next saw him in the outpatient clinic about a month later, he looked perfectly normal: he was wearing a dark blue suit, was extremely well groomed, and radiated happiness to friends and strangers alike. Some of those strangers were other patients and their families, and they, in turn, took hope. We were elated, and I called the ward nurses to come down to see Sam in the clinic. We all needed that kind of positive reinforcement.

Although I soon left the Leukemia Service, and later the National Cancer Institute, Sam sent me cards periodically for perhaps three years, until his disease recurred. It eventually killed him, because it had become resistant to the chemotherapy. But those cards never failed to mention his enormous joy of having made the "right" decision to persevere. To me, Sam was a hero—as were the many others through the years, children and adults alike, who courageously faced this dreadful foe.

PART I

A Disease of Despair

Maria

Würzberg, Germany, 1860 (based on the original case report).

It was the third day in a row that Maria had come home from kindergarten without a gold or silver star. More bothersome to her mother was the teacher's neatly written note saying that the five-year-old girl was not paying attention to her assignments or to her choral singing. Maria had been doing well in her report cards in this second year of kindergarten, and she was the pride of her parents. But now Maria herself seemed listless and uncommunicative. Mama Speyer resolved to talk with the teacher the next day.

As the mother bathed her two daughters that night, she was alarmed to see the red splotches over Maria's skin—her upper arms, legs, and trunk had new marks. But the most noticeable marks looked like blood blisters over both buttocks. Maria admitted that the teacher had given her some lashes with a switch, but she didn't understand why. The other children had laughed at her while she cried, and she had been ashamed. Mama Speyer was overwhelmed with fear and confusion. Her husband was employed on a carpentry job outside of the city and would not return until the next night. He had taken the family horse-drawn cart to transport himself and the tools of his craft.

Maria did not go to school the next day. Instead, both she and her younger sister Eva were taken to the family doctor who had delivered them. Until recently Mama had been more concerned about Eva, because the three-year-old had not eaten normally or played with her usual vigor for several weeks. Mama Speyer had been planning to have the doctor check her when the more urgent problem of Maria arose on the previous day. Mama was now pregnant with her sixth child—the third by this marriage to Hans Speyer. Two of her three children by her first husband had died between the ages of one and three. The causes of death were not known.

Herr Doctor Stern was always cheerful with the girls and even allowed them to listen to his elegant gold vest pocket timepiece. He examined each child in turn, palpating gently here and there and listening to the front and back of the chest by putting his cold ear to their warm skin. When he did that, he tickled them with his beard and made them laugh. Dr. Stern told the anxious mother that both children were suffering from pallor and asthenia, or loss of strength. He was most concerned about the many "blood spots" on Maria's skin; indeed, new bruises had occurred since the previous day. Both Maria and Eva were found to have enlarged spleens (milztumoren), but Maria's spleen was huge, taking up most of the left side of the abdomen. Stern thought a new sort of fever must have affected the spleen. Since he believed it was contagious, he ordered the children to stay at home and prescribed cod liver oil and other purgative medicines for them.

Eva improved, but her sister did not. Within two days the doctor had to make a house call because Maria was much worse—she was hot, irritable, and more bruised. The purgatives had taken their toll, for her skin was dry and flaky, her eyes were sunken in their sockets, and she was too weak to arise from the bed. Maria had no desire to listen to the timepiece when it was offered, and she did not give her customary laugh when examined. Eva was feeling better; she was too exuberant to sit still during the doctor's visit. Dr. Stern told both parents that he had not had a case like Maria's before and he would consult with Dr. Biermer, a man who traveled widely to medical meetings and was an expert diagnostician.

The child slept for long stretches of the day and night and was extremely irritable when awake. Her head hurt and her neck was stiff. Papa Speyer fashioned a wooden funnel with a fine spout to give her milk and soup, since she was unable to sit up on her own. Biermer arrived the next day to examine Maria. He then consulted with Dr. Stern and left in his buggy to get more instruments, refusing to speak to the parents until his examination was completed. When he returned, he drew a blood sample with a superficial scalpel cut on the forearm. Maria cried briefly because taking the sample woke her up. The good doctor went to examine the blood under a new device called a microscope, while Mama pressed a handkerchief tightly against the bleeding wound.

Papa Speyer helped the doctor set the delicate instrument on a shelf near the best-lit window in the house. A candle was placed so that its light was reflected via a mirror through the lenses, so the doctor could see the structure of Maria's blood. The examination was repeated as the doctor first grunted his disapproval and then exulted at his success. After a private conference with Dr. Stern, who took his turn at squinting through the single eyepiece of the microscope, Dr. Biermer next ushered in the trembling Speyer parents.

They only half heard the litany of findings about Maria—anemia, asthenia, an enlarged heart, possible pneumonia, a hugely enlarged spleen and liver, and hemorrhages in the skin. The doctor excitedly explained that a similar illness, invariably fatal, had been described in the late 1840s and termed *Leukamie* ("white blood")—but it had never been reported in a child before. This was the very first case and Biermer would report it to the Academy "after she dies—and we are able to do a complete examination."

Herr Doctor Stern tended to Mama Speyer, who had fainted, and Papa tried to calm the screaming Eva, while Maria slept in the next room. If the doctors understood the cruelty of what they had just said, they showed no sign of it—they had done what they perceived to be their professional duty. They departed together, deeply involved in an animated discussion of this extraordinary *exquisiten Fall von Leukamie* (exquisite case of leukemia) in a child. From the doorstep, Hans Speyer called his thanks to the doctors for their work—he thought that he and his wife owed these learned men that, despite the gravity of the news.

Late that afternoon, Maria cried out in her sleep. Then she vomited bright reddish stomach contents halfway across the room. It gushed and spurted from her mouth, and, as the flow lessened, some dribbled from her lips. (This would later be called projectile vomiting; in such cases it generally signifies an increase in pressure in the brain—such as from hemorrhage or a tumor.) By the time the doctor returned, the child lay dead in a clean white bed. Mama Speyer had washed her and placed her in their finest starched sheets. Dr. Stern solemnly made the arrangements for an autopsy.

CHAPTER 1

The Discovery of Leukemia

Life is short, the art long, the occasion fleeting, experience fallacious and judgment difficult.

—*Hippocrates*

Maria's brief illness and death went down in medical history because hers was the first case of childhood leukemia to be described. But the history of cancer is as old as humanity: the bones of some early humans reveal unmistakable signs of cancer. The great physician-healers of classical antiquity, Hippocrates and Galen, carefully described cases of cancer in their patients, hypothesized about cancer's cause, and tried to find ways to treat it.

If the ancient doctors saw cases of leukemia (and it is reasonable to assume they did), they did not describe it clearly or give it a special name. The naming of the disease and the recognition of its cancerous character required over two thousand years of anatomical studies, a major shift in the way health and disease were explained, and a set of technologies that made it possible to see blood cells and the tissues that generated them. These three developments converged in the mid-nineteenth century, and all were prerequisites to recognizing the very existence of childhood leukemia as a distinct disease entity and to homing in on its essential character as a malignancy of the blood-forming tissues in children and adults.

Nineteenth-century physicians inherited a long tradition of ascribing melancholy and peevishness to "an attack of the spleen," so it is not surprising that they would take note of patients whose spleens were enormously enlarged. The physicians reported that such patients were often very pale and weak, had enlarged glands in the neck, armpits, and groin, and bruised easily. Dr. Richard Bright of Guy's Hospital and Physician

Extraordinary to Queen Victoria took a special interest in the function and diseases of the spleen. In 1838 he wrote perspicaciously, as C. C. Sturgis notes, "With regard to the function of the spleen, we have every reason to believe that it affords important assistance in repairing the blood." He described alterations in the spleen, including congestion, hardening, softening, inflammation, gangrene, and tuberculosis. He drew attention to a condition he had seen in a number of patients: "Fleshy hardness with enlargement, in which the spleen often obtains prodigious size, filling up the whole left side of the abdomen. It is astonishing with what rapidity this enormous growth takes place. In young children this form of the disease is still more frequent than in adults and with them it is more fatal. It often begins to show itself at two to three months of age and such children seldom live above a year, or two or three." Although Bright never examined the blood of these patients, he intuitively deduced that the enlargement of the spleen was somehow the result of a disease originating elsewhere in the body and the blood: "I may observe generally in reference to splenic disease that it is probable that the spleen is greatly influenced by the derangement of many of the other organs of the body. We cannot doubt that whatever acts on the circulating system must in some degree influence the spleen: which obviously, from its structure and appearance, receives large quantities of blood."

In their careful review of the history of leukemia, Dr. Frederick Gunz and Dr. E. S. Henderson conclude that the first accurate description of a case of leukemia was made in 1827 by Alfred Velpeau. This French physician had been caring for a sixty-three-year-old patient, a florist who also sold lemonade on the side, but "who had abandoned himself to the abuse of spirituous liquor and of women, without, however, becoming syphilitic." (That alone was noteworthy in those days.) This man became ill with a swelling in the abdomen, fever, and weakness, and he died soon after admission to the hospital. At the time of the autopsy, he was found to have an enormous liver and spleen—the latter weighing some 10 pounds, which would be large for a newborn baby, let alone a spleen. The blood had a peculiar appearance, "like gruel . . . resembling in consistency and color the yeast of red wine . . . one might have asked if it were not rather laudable pus, mixed with the blackish coloring matter, than blood." It was this remarkable appearance of the blood that also attracted the attention of other physicians when they saw subsequent cases. Of course,

Velpeau did not know what it was that he was describing—his patient's malady was nameless. Still, he created a record that guided others.

The disease was first recognized in France by Doctors Barth and Donne when, in 1839, Barth studied a forty-four-year-old Parisian woman who had enlargement of the spleen. After she died, the postmortem examination revealed the blood to have a puslike appearance. The microscopic study carried out by Dr. Donne showed that more than half the blood cells were "white globules" of the type described by Dr. William Hewson in 1774. (The microscope had been in scientific use since 1614, but had not been used to describe blood diseases prior to the 1830s.) Although Barth's 1839 patient study was not published until 1856, Donne had published a monograph in 1844 which referred to this and several such patients who may well have had leukemia. Others may equally well have died of infection, however, for the records are unclear. In 1845 several cases of leukemia, which presented clinical, autopsy, and microscopic findings, were simultaneously published in Edinburgh and Berlin. In the Edinburgh case, Dr. David Craigie described a patient who, at the time of autopsy, was found to have a greatly enlarged spleen and liver with generalized glandular enlargement, and blood that showed "globules of purulent matter (pus)." Craigie failed to appreciate the significance of his findings and might never have published the case, had he not attended his colleague's postmortem examination of a second, similar case.

When Dr. John Hughes Bennett saw a remarkable patient in Scotland in 1845, he commented on the outstanding similarity between his case and that reported by Dr. Craigie.

> John Menteith, age 28, a slater, married, admitted into the clinical ward of the Royal Infirmary, February 27, 1845. He is of dark complexion, usually healthy and temperate; states that twenty months ago he was affected with great listlessness on exertion, which has continued to this time. In June last he noticed a tumour in the left side of the abdomen, which has gradually increased in size till four months since, when it became stationary. [This would signify his large spleen.]
>
> It was never painful till last week, after the application of three blisters to it. [Doctors would use a poultice dressing to apply a highly irritating chemical to the skin in order to cause a chemical burn and blistering of the area, thinking that the tissues below would be more likely to heal.] Since then several other small tumours have appeared in his neck, armpits, and groins, at first attended with a sharp pain, which has now, however,

disappeared from all of them. Before he noticed the tumour he had frequent vomiting in the morning. The bowels are usually constipated, appetite good, is not subject to indigestion, had no vomiting since he noticed the tumour. Has used chiefly purgative medicines, especially croton oil, has employed friction with a liniment, and had the tumour blistered.

Bennett goes on to report further medical details, but in essence the patient developed fever, thirst, and diarrhea and died suddenly two weeks later. Doctors did a careful autopsy, examined the organs in great detail, and remarked on the huge enlargement of the liver (11 pounds) and spleen (8 pounds). The most striking finding, and one that they could not correctly explain, was the appearance of the blood. When they opened the cavities of the heart and large veins, they found that the clotted blood had separated into a brick-red lower portion and a yellow upper portion that "resembled thick creamy pus." And yet with pus they would have expected to find a local infection—but none was found. They did do microscopy studies to show "colorless globules" in the top portion, but did not appreciate the fact that the cells were not the normal type of white blood cells that one would find with infection. These were actually leukemic cells, a previously undescribed form of cancer involving cells of the white blood cell variety. Bennett looked and wondered, but in the end he concluded that "pus in the blood was the cause of death." Thus did discovery of this new disease elude Bennett as well.

In 1845, only months after Bennett's encounter with the disease, the great German pathologist Dr. Rudolf Virchow published a similar case, and it was he who really recognized its unique nature. Both of these cases were published within a month of each other, both had the appearance of pus in the blood, and, in the Virchow case, there were relatively few red corpuscles and many colorless or white corpuscles. Because of the reversed relationship between red and white blood cells as compared with normal blood, Virchow used the term "white blood" (*weisses blut*), or leukemia, to describe this illness.

Bennett thought the term leukemia was a misnomer; indeed they argued over it for years. But in the end, he did accept Virchow's interpretation of the nature of the disease and withdrew his former idea that it was an infection in the blood.

In all the initial cases of leukemia described by Barth and Donne, Craigie, Bennett, and Virchow, the disease was recognized only at the time of autopsy. The ability to establish a diagnosis in this way obviously cannot endear the doctor to his patients, for it can never lead to an effective treatment. Still, it was an important step, for it showed what might be found during life *if* the proper tests were done.

Leukemia in a living person was first recognized in 1845 in a patient cared for by Dr. Nairne in London, although he incorrectly identified it at the time. He and a Dr. Henry Fuller reported that the blood of this patient examined during life, and again after death, showed on each occasion a very large number of these colorless globules, or white blood cells. At autopsy there was massive enlargement of the liver and spleen, just as with the other cases that had been reported. They initially believed that this disease was caused by exposure to malaria, but still it was the first account of a case of leukemia diagnosed during life. Soon thereafter, recognition of the disease became common, including Biermer's first published record (1861) of leukemia occurring in a child, our friend Maria. He noted her extreme pallor and the great enlargement of her liver, spleen, and lymph glands. Biermer established the diagnosis, but could do nothing but watch the child slide rapidly downhill and die. Autopsy confirmed the findings of huge spleen and liver, and revealed the enlargement of the heart.

In reconstructing the events surrounding the recognition of leukemia, it seems that there was considerable argument by the experts of the time as to whether this condition was infectious or not, an issue that took years to unravel. It was again Virchow who, in 1856, published a paper stating that the colorless (or white) corpuscles or cells were always present in normal blood and in most inflammatory conditions, and that an increase in the number of white cells was not sufficient to characterize the leukemia—in which there was also an important decrease in the number of normal red corpuscles and serious changes in certain organs, such as the liver and the spleen.

As additional patients were being described by other doctors, it was increasingly the opinion that the increased number of white corpuscles was not due to an inflammation or infection. Nonetheless, at a major medical meeting in Paris in 1855, there were still those who failed to recognize leukemia as a distinct entity, including one physician who told his learned colleagues that "leukemia has no special causes, special symptoms, particular anatomic lesions, or specific treatment, and I thus conclude that it does not exist as a distinct malady." This ostrichlike view was expanded by another physician who added, "There are enough diseases without inventing any new ones." Perhaps resistance of this type serves a useful function in that it may stimulate restless adventurers to reach new heights of accomplishment.

For nearly twenty centuries the theory of humoral pathology influenced the ideas of medical people, at least until Giovanni Morgagni (1761) and Xavier Bichat (1800) asserted that humoral imbalances do not influence the whole body and that disease occurs in specific organs where illnesses originate, as in the liver, heart, kidneys, and so on. It remained for Virchow (1855) to show that it is cells that give rise to other cells, which in turn aggregate to form tissues and organs, something that every youngster learns in school today. His classic work on cellular pathology laid the foundation for both biology and pathology.

Although medicine in Germany in the mid–nineteenth century was at a very low level compared with France, Virchow helped to change that situation remarkably by his own research, productivity, and leadership over a period of fifty years. Virchow established that the cell—not one of the so-called basic fluids or humors, nor even the amorphous germinal elements proposed by scholars of the previous hundred years—is the fundamental unit in which disease occurs. Cancer comes from cells, and the type of cancer that develops depends on the constitutional or hereditary predisposition of the patient and on the nature of the irritating stimulus (which we now call a chemical or viral carcinogen).

Virchow's work in biochemistry and microscopy gave him the tools to see a new world of cells, and he exhorted his students to "learn to see microscopically." Everything Virchow did was done with enormous conviction. In 1845 he began publishing papers on leukemia and went on to write classic works about cancer, infections, nerves, and general pathology. He was a passionate man in his personal life, too, criticizing his government, fighting at the barricades when revolution broke out in Berlin in 1848, and challenging the Aryan anthropological theories propounded by a former student. After he was elected to the Prussian legislature, he led a desperate fight against the dictatorship of Otto von Bismarck. The latter became so annoyed with this renowned scientist turned statesman that he challenged him to a duel. Fortunately, this never came to pass.

Somehow, in the midst of all his political and scientific activities, Virchow found time to distinguish the two major kinds of leukemia. He recognized that the splenic, or *myelogenous*, kind revealed itself initially or mainly in the spleen. The *lymphatic* kind, by contrast, seemed especially to involve the lymph glands (in the neck, groin, and armpits). But even with the microscope he could not determine whether the white blood cells he saw accumulating in the two kinds of leukemia were identical to the white blood cells in the blood of normal, healthy people.

The next critical step in understanding leukemia came with a new technique for marking and differentiating cells. In 1890, while still a student, Paul Ehrlich—another great German scientist—discovered that, by staining cells with various aniline dyes, he could distinguish among kinds of cells and even see previously invisible structures inside the cells. This made it possible to see that there was more than one kind of white blood cell. In fact, there were many different kinds—although it would take many more years to realize that each kind had its own special job in the body, that each kind could become malignant and thus give rise to a particular kind of leukemia. By 1877 scientists had identified *myeloid* white blood cells, which originate in the marrow of bones (the Greek word *myelos* meant both bone marrow and spinal cord) and play a crucial role in the body's response to infection. The new stains stuck to tiny granules inside these myeloid cells and made the cells easy to spot when a blood sample was examined under the microscope. The myeloid cells turned out to be the white blood cells that, if they became malignant, were characteristic of Virchow's splenic or myelogenous leukemia: generated in the bone marrow, but invading the liver and spleen (and other organs and tissues).

Virchow's other kind of leukemia, lymphatic leukemia, was harder to match up with a particular kind of white blood cell. As careful microscopy eventually showed, the white blood cells characteristic of this kind of leukemia, the lymphocytes, lacked the easily stained granules. The lymphocytes originated not just in the bone marrow but in the spleen and—as their name implies—in the lymph nodes. Like the myeloid cells, they could migrate to any other organ or tissue. In healthy bodies, the lymphocytes regulate the body's immune response, chiefly by making antibodies. In lymphatic leukemia—or lymphocytic leukemia, as it was eventually renamed—these critical white blood cells lost their normal ability to mount an immune response and multiplied so uncontrollably that they swamped all other white and red blood cells.

17

The drive to classify different kinds of leukemias continued throughout the nineteenth and twentieth centuries. Increasing technical sophistication made it possible to see subclasses of the various kinds of blood cells—and their corresponding leukemias. One kind originates in the cells that make platelets, the tiny white blood cells that normally plug up broken blood vessels in wounds and bruises. Another, quite unexpected kind arises in the precursors of *red* blood cells (erythrocytes) in the bone marrow, producing the paradoxically named erythroleukemia: "red white-blood."

Physicians noticed that some forms of leukemia were much more aggressive than others. The *acute leukemias* killed quickly, while *chronic leukemias* might allow three to ten or more years of life. Both the myelogenous and lymphatic leukemias had their acute and chronic forms.

Differences among the kinds of victims were also categorized. Mid-nineteenth-century scientists detected leukemias in animals as well as humans: Dr. Leisering first recognized the disease in horses in 1858, and in pigs in 1865. Soon thereafter it was discovered in birds, cows, mice, cats, and other animals. (Although study of these animal leukemias was very important for understanding the course of the disease in humans, there was a major difference: apparently only a few, very rare human leukemias are caused by viruses, whereas most animal leukemias are viral.) Among humans, Bright's original insight was confirmed: different groups of people were apt to get different kinds of leukemia. Chronic lymphatic leukemia (CLL) was most often found in older adults; acute myelogenous leukemia (AML) in young adults. Acute lymphocytic leukemia (ALL), characterized by the uncontrollably rapid growth of primitive lymphatic cells and the invasion of normal organs (such as the liver and brain), so often struck children under eighteen that it became commonly known as childhood leukemia—even though many adults were its victims too. (We are experiencing about 28,000 new cases of leukemia each year in the United States, about half acute and half chronic: 2,000 new cases of childhood ALL are included in this figure.)

The two forms of acute leukemia, lymphocytic and myelogenous, do similar damage to their victims. Patients with acute lymphocytic leukemia bleed easily, become covered with bruises as tiny injured blood vessels leak under the skin, and sometimes scream with pain from the pressure of leukemic cells multiplying within the bone marrow cavity. Septicemia—because there are not enough normal white blood cells to fight infection—

and bleeding into the brain become life-threatening problems. The torment is much the same for patients with acute myelogenous leukemia.

The tricky work of figuring out the confusing array of leukemias had, at the time, no practical clinical importance. It gave physicians plenty to wrangle over at medical meetings and encouraged them to make closer observations of leukemic patients, but it did not help their patients at all. No matter how well the doctors could diagnose the particular kind of leukemia in each case, they could do nothing except wait for the inevitable outcome. Everyone with leukemia died from it, unless some accident or other illness carried them off first. No wonder only a handful of physicians and researchers persisted in studying leukemia, trying to find a clue that might lead to a cure.

The search for a cure for leukemia first looked for inspiration to the triumphs over infectious disease in the late nineteenth century and early twentieth century. It did not matter that leukemia was not transmitted from person to person. That fact was established in the early days of American leukemia research when researchers injected prisoner-volunteers with billions of leukemic cells and found that, fortunately, none of the inmates contracted the disease. (Such a desperate experiment on humans was criticized at the time and would be absolutely forbidden today as dangerous and unethical.)

In particular, researchers looked at the possibility that chemotherapy—the use of biochemically potent drugs—could beat cancer and leukemia as it had beaten infectious diseases. The instinct was sound: ultimately this line of work was very fruitful. It had a long history behind it. The chemical treatment of cancer goes back to the first century of the modern era when crocus extracts—long afterwards shown to contain the potent mutagen colchicine—were used on local cancers. During the Renaissance, remedies based on arsenic, mercury, bismuth, antimony, silver, copper, and zinc entered the physician's arsenal. None of these had any effect on cancer, although much later, in the 1860s, there was a brief flurry of optimism over potassium arsenate, which seemed to help chronic leukemia and lymphoma temporarily. But this led nowhere. Joseph Burchenal points to quinine as the first persuasive example of a chemical that was effective against a specific infectious disease, malaria.

Gradually other drugs based on chemical dyes and toxic compounds were developed to treat such widespread infectious diseases as malaria and trypanosomiasis. These drugs were, however, effective only against specific kinds of microorganisms: trypanosomas, spirochetes (the cause of syphilis), and parasites such as plasmodium infections that cause malaria. Infections caused by bacteria still seemed impossible to cure. The experts of the day felt sure that it was utterly impossible to kill the bacteria without killing the patient as well.

The first trickle of hope that cancer too might be cured by chemotherapy came, ironically, out of the most terrible use of the chemists' art: chemical warfare.

Paul Ehrlich had, in the course of his investigations of the biological effects of all kinds of chemical compounds, discovered a group of highly reactive derivatives of extracts from mustard plants and noted the complex toxic properties of nitrogen mustard and related alkylating agents. Other German chemists continued to study these compounds and came up with mustard gas, the horrifying new weapon of World War I. Mustard gas did not become a major weapon in "the war to end all wars," but only because the German generals could not command the winds. They could not stop the clouds of poisonous gas from being blown back on their own lines. Many soldiers on both sides were injured or died from exposure to the gas.

Trying to understand the specific effects of mustard gas, the military physicians did autopsies on its victims. Researchers also studied the effects of exposing dogs and other animals to these compounds. They observed that it severely damaged the bone marrow and lymph nodes—precisely (though they did not say so) the sites affected in many cancers and leukemias.

These wartime findings were published in 1919, but remained unnoticed until the chemical studies were resumed during World War II, this time by the Allies. Could this damaging effect against normal lymph nodes be used against cancerous nodes? Studies with nitrogen mustard at Yale in 1942 showed shrinkage of lymphoma in mice, followed by the striking improvement of a treated patient. This was then extended by a talented group of scientists assembled for the war effort at Edgewood Arsenal, Maryland, and by clinical studies done in Salt Lake City and elsewhere.

On the other side of the Atlantic, a London team at the Chester Beatty Institute headed up by Alexander Haddow was synthesizing other mustard derivatives such as urethane and, later, chlorambucil and busulfan, which became mainstays in the management of chronic forms of leukemia. Although such drugs are very important in cancer chemotherapy, they are not central to the cure of acute leukemia except as the intellectual beginnings for many of the key participants in that story.

Meanwhile, the record of endless defeat, the inevitable fatality of leukemia, meant that a large part of the medical profession chose to concentrate on other diseases, ones that offered some hope of recovery for their patients. There were, however, notable exceptions, whom we shall meet.

CHAPTER 2

Plans without Blueprints

Science is built up with facts, as a house is with stones. But a collection of facts is no more a science than a heap of stones is a house.

—Jules Henri Poincaré

There was no definitive starting point in the search for a cure to childhood leukemia, no finish line to indicate success. When success did come, it was a great surprise. Even the doctors who were doing the clinical studies could not believe that they had succeeded in curing children.

Perhaps it should not have been a surprise. In retrospect, it does not seem so complicated—but then, neither does atomic energy. Any first-class graduate student in physics today can pull it off, but it took the leading minds in physics to orchestrate the Manhattan Project during World War II and demonstrate the power of the atom. The four-minute mile—once thought the fundamental limit to human speed—is now broken by outstanding high school runners. Accomplishments that once seemed impossible become commonplace with the passage of time. All it takes, apparently, is the breaking of that first barrier.

Medical discoveries have traditionally been the product of discoveries by a scientist working alone on a unique project (as with William Jenner and the discovery of vaccination against smallpox) or racing in competition with others to be the first (as with the discovery of insulin to control diabetes). While the quest to cure childhood leukemia has some of the elements of both these traditions, it may have been the first example of a major, quasi-national cooperative effort among scientists to cure a specific disease. Thus it marks a new era in medical research: the first use of carefully controlled clinical trials and the first deliberate use of chemicals to cure a pervasive malignancy. Although it did not start out as a coordinated effort—indeed, no one could possibly have predicted who or what talents would be essential to the team—it could not have been done alone. The solution required many different ideas, drugs, medical concepts, means of treating infection and bleeding, the sum of which was far beyond the scope of any individual scientist or institution.

There was no master blueprint for finding a cure for leukemia, only the determination to find a way to end the suffering and a willingness to look for even tiny gains that might yield ideas for further progress. A baseball fan would call it a game won by base hits, not home runs. Strangest of all, no one recognized the moment when victory was at hand. No one can say truthfully, in this year we conquered leukemia, or this was the first patient cured of leukemia. It was difficult to tell the difference between a prolonged remission, in which a person would look perfectly well but would eventually relapse and die, and a permanent cure. Despite the vagueness of the beginning and the close of the story, this is a noble chapter in American medicine that is now ready to be told.

This series of mixed metaphors—race, blueprint, stepping stone, ball-game, battle—is indicative of the patchwork quilt that had to be pieced together to solve so enormous and complex a medical problem. Scientists had no known cause, no cure, and a very long list of ways a child might die from leukemia. How were they to know where to begin to look for an answer? The solution came from the combined efforts of chemists, biologists, clinical researchers, blood bank experts, infectious disease specialists, and research scientists who were willing to tackle small problems as a means to an end. They had no guarantees that their hard work would be rewarded; indeed, conventional wisdom told them they were fools to work so hard on something so obviously fruitless.

To many scientists and doctors in the first couple of decades of the twentieth century, the most interesting new development in medicine was the elucidation of nutritional deficiency diseases. The startling discovery of vitamins' crucial role in the maintenance of health and the dire consequences—scurvy, beriberi, rickets—of a lack of tiny amounts of these mysterious chemicals suggested a new approach to curing cancer. Perhaps the rapidly growing cells of cancers had special nutritional requirements. If so, perhaps they could be starved into submission. The idea was worth a closer look.

At Mount Sinai Hospital in New York, in an unventilated basement laboratory, one group of researchers set to work in 1938 to investigate the possibility. My own initiation into cancer research began there as a young boy, helping my father. My father, Daniel Laszlo, was a Viennese physician with a specialty in cardiac physiology who had brought our family to New York to escape the impending war in Europe. He accepted a research position at Mount Sinai in a lab nominally headed by a genial, independently wealthy surgeon, Richard Lewisohn, who came in occasionally to see what was happening.

My father and two other talented refugee scientists, Rudolf and Cecilie Leuchtenberger, began an intensive study of the role of nutritional factors in cancer. The first step was to work out a system for reproducing cancer at will in mice.

They transplanted tumors by injecting live cancer cells into mice and making daily measurements of the size of the growing tumors. By measuring the rates of growth, they standardized their system so that they could determine with confidence whether tumors were shrinking under the influence of the experimental treatments.

I remember vividly how much labor went into caring for the hundreds of mice. When the animal caretaker was off duty on weekends, my father would take me along to help clean the cages and give the mice their water and special diets. I learned how to keep the labels, mice, and cages from getting mixed up. I mastered the trick of twisting a moistened glass tube into the cork or rubber stopper of a water bottle, and then tipping the bottle upside down so the water would fill the tube, yet not spill out. I would watch the mouse lift its head to drink, almost like a baby at a bottle, but licking rather than sucking at the water.

It was remarkable that in some of the cages the tumors were almost as large as the mice that were dragging them along. By this point, the animals would be listless, their fur ruffled, and we would know that they were within a day or two of death. In other cages, tumors inoculated at the same time were much smaller, the animals looked healthier and more alert, and were feeding.

As each mouse died, it was weighed and carefully autopsied. The tumor was examined, measured, and then fixed in a formalin solution so that it could be processed for microscopic analysis. It was an unpleasant business to pick out the stiff mouse, stretch it out on its back, pin down the four paws to a board, and begin the dissection. I watched this part of the process, staying back a few feet to avoid the fetid odor once the abdominal cavity was opened. The tumors were carefully dissected out and weighed, as were normal organs like the liver and spleen.

Something other than the unpleasant smell of those mice hung about us in the air. There was a sense of excitement that filled that laboratory almost to the point of disbelief.

My father and his colleagues were finding that mice fed with certain enriched extracts of yeast and barley and other natural products escaped death from cancer: the tumors stopped growing. Yet when the team tried to isolate the tumor-stopping substance, they got exciting but confusing results. Some extracts seemed to do exactly the opposite of what the researchers expected: instead of inhibiting tumor growth, these substances promoted the growth of the tumors. No one else had ever been able to use natural substances to make tumors grow or shrink in animals. What were the substances responsible for this, and was this a phenomenon that could be reproduced in people who had cancer? More and more nutrients were tested from various sources, and on several occasions I accompanied my father to breweries to obtain different specimens of yeast.

More mice and supplies were required in order to continue the research, and my father appealed to his superiors for an additional two thousand dollars. Uncertain of the importance of the work, the laboratory director at Mount Sinai called in Dr. C. P. Rhoads, director of Memorial Sloan-Kettering Cancer Center. Independent tests were run by a prominent cancer researcher from that institute. Dr. Sugiura was unable to cause his mouse tumors (a different strain—of both mice and kinds of tumor—than used at Mount Sinai) to shrink with the dietary program provided by the Laszlo-Leuchtenberger team, and the advice given to the Mount Sinai administrators was not to put any more money into the project. When my father pleaded with the director for the additional funds, he was told, "Laszlo, when you cure your first cancer patient, then I'll give you the money." My father's response was automatic: "When I cure my first cancer patient, I won't have to come to you for money."

Ironically, when Babe Ruth was dying of cancer at Mount Sinai, hospital officials and Dr. Lewisohn arranged for him to receive the extracts that my father's laboratory had been testing in mice—the very work these administrators would not support with additional funds. My father was horrified, since the extracts had not been adequately tested in animals, had never been given to humans, and had the potential to make the Babe worse.

25

On September 5, 1947, Dr. Lewisohn reported to the Fourth International Cancer Research Congress meeting in St. Louis the remarkable research advance in prolonging the life and easing the pain of an unnamed fifty-two-year-old man with cancer of the nasal passages, face, and neck. This report in fact referred to Babe Ruth, who had entered Mount Sinai in June 1947 with excruciating pain and inability to eat despite surgery and radiation treatments. After six weeks of injections of folic acid derivatives called pteropterins, as prepared by Lederle Laboratories, the cancer shrank and the patient was improved. Although clearly not a cure, this very preliminary report raised considerable excitement in the medical world. The story was never written up in the literature, and I doubt that there will ever be an authoritative account of this unusual beginning to the metabolic treatment of cancer.

My father was so upset that he resigned from Mount Sinai and moved to Montefiore Hospital, where he began the Neoplastic Disease Service, the first cancer service of its kind in a general hospital. Disenchanted with the Mount Sinai experience, he never again worked on nutritional factors in cancer and switched to the new area of using radioisotopes to study bone metabolism. The Leuchtenbergers also moved on to distinguished careers in other areas of science. The premature termination of the program left many unanswered questions about the nature of the substances that were involved and why the work was not reproducible at Memorial.

Despite the doubts of the Memorial Sloan-Kettering researchers about the work in that smelly Mount Sinai basement, something about the project continued to tantalize scientists. The idea that a nutritional factor, or a chemical variation of it, could somehow affect the growth of cancerous cells turned out to be the first successful step in the cure of leukemia.

The first fruits of the new research were reported in a landmark paper, "Temporary Remissions in Acute Leukemia in Children Prolonged by Folic Acid Antagonist, 4-Aminopteroylglutamic Acid (Aminopterin)" in the *New England Journal of Medicine* in 1948: Sidney Farber, Louis Diamond, and colleagues at Boston's Children's Hospital said they had obtained remissions in leukemia patients by administering a new drug called aminopterin. The paper was the first tangible evidence that scientists could create chemicals that would alter the course of this disease, for the remarkable thing about aminopterin was that it had been specially designed to do this.

Dr. Sidney Farber died without ever explaining why he decided to pursue a lead that he himself had declared a blind alley. So, rather than devoting a whole chapter to his work as I do with other major contributors to leukemia research, I can only give the outlines of what he accomplished. Farber's name and work will come up over and over again in the following chapters as a champion of the effort to cure leukemia.

Farber knew about my father's and the Leuchtenbergers' work. It had stimulated the doubters at Memorial Sloan-Kettering to try some experiments of their own with nutritional factors on tumor growth. When they were unable to confirm antitumor activity, Farber evidently advised them to give it up and stop wasting their time. Yet he himself began to undertake some experiments with the nutritional factor that, in 1941, had been named folic acid.

The existence of folic acid had been strongly suggested by Dr. Lucy Wills's studies of tropical anemia in the 1930s. She and her colleagues had shown that women in India had a form of anemia that would, like pernicious anemia, get better when they ate liver and crude extracts of liver. The purified liver extracts that cured pernicious anemia, however, did not help against tropical anemia: in the process of purifying the extract the so-called Wills Factor was being lost. The factor that cured tropical anemia, folic acid, was actually first isolated from leafy vegetables (and took its name from the Latin name for "leaf," *folium*).

Once folic acid was isolated, research on its precise structure and function was possible. In 1945 chemists realized that, structurally, folic acid was a member of a class of chemical compounds, pteridines, that are very common in all sorts of living tissues. (Pteridines get their name from the Greek word for "wing" because they, among other things, provide the colorful pigments in butterfly wings.)

Functionally, folic acid is an important growth factor in cells, and especially in blood cells—the cells most affected by leukemia. Without folic acid, neither normal nor cancerous cells can make DNA or divide. Interfering in the cancer cell's use of folic acid to reproduce thus seemed as if it might be one way to reverse the growth of tumors and the multiplication of leukemic cells. The picture was complicated, however, by the fact that related pteridines seemed to have the opposite effect on cells and tumors. Much later, scientists realized that the balance between folic acid and its pteridine "cousins" dictated whether animal tumors would grow or shrink (the full scientific details are still not sorted out).

Farber, for reasons that are not recorded and certainly not obvious, began to treat twelve leukemia patients in Children's Hospital with folic acid. He knew so little about it at the time that he called my father to ask more about their work and even how to spell folic acid. He concluded that giving folic acid made matters worse, not better, for these patients.

Although most experts believe that his conclusion about the harmfulness of folic acid to children with progressive acute leukemia was probably erroneous (the scientific issues remain somewhat unclear), the pharmaceutical chemists at Lederle and American Cyanamid believed him and came up with a brilliant idea: if folic acid made leukemia worse, they argued, why not design a chemical compound that would look a lot like folic acid to the leukemic cells but would block their activity? That is, why not create an *antagonist* to folic acid? The result was a new compound called aminopterin.

The outcome was striking: aminopterin did bring about remissions. True, the remissions were brief and only occurred in some patients, yet never before had anyone succeeded in even doing that. Farber's 1948 report in the *New England Journal of Medicine* triggered the search for other antagonists to folic acid. Within a year, methotrexate was synthesized. This close variation on folic acid soon became the most widely used of the folic acid derivatives against acute leukemia and many other cancers.

Now let me introduce the scientists whose intertwined lives and work form the heart of this book.

To start off, I use—as a surrogate for Sidney Farber—his early collaborator, Dr. Donald Pinkel. Pinkel's recollections of the early years of leukemia research give a vivid picture of what it was like to see those first promising results with aminopterin and methotrexate in the late 1940s and the bitterness of not being able to do more to save patients at that time.

The story then moves to Dr. Joseph Burchenal at Memorial Sloan-Kettering Cancer Center in New York, who saw with his own astonished eyes what Farber had accomplished in Boston and decided to start working on folic acid antagonists himself. He and his able co-workers set about testing one inhibitor after another, looking for some sign of therapeutic effectiveness in tumor-bearing mice. Whenever they found a lead, they would try to exploit it to help their patients in the hospital.

Supplying Burchenal with a stream of ever-more sophisticated chemical compounds were two pharmaceutical chemists at the Burroughs Well-

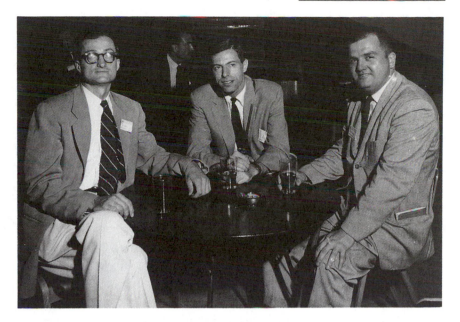

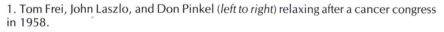

1. Tom Frei, John Laszlo, and Don Pinkel (*left to right*) relaxing after a cancer congress in 1958.

come Company: George Hitchings, Ph.D., and his young assistant, Gertrude Elion. Hitchings and Elion very deliberately and effectively set themselves the task of synthesizing and testing new classes of drugs that would interfere with the normal metabolism of cells. They focused especially on drugs that would wreck the metabolism of nucleic acid—years before the genetic code embodied in the nucleic acids was discovered. As important as the drugs they designed was their system for testing the drugs: Hitchings developed simple bacterial metabolic systems to detect precisely which metabolic process a chemical compound was promoting or blocking. In 1951 the most promising antimetabolite drug for leukemia to come out of Hitchings and Elion's lab—6-mercaptopurine, or 6-MP, for short—was (like the folic acid antagonists before it) immediately tested on children with leukemia in Burchenal's hospital. (Today, government regulations concerning clinical trials of new drugs would require much more extensive testing on animals first.)

The hopes that were raised by the remissions Burchenal obtained with Hitchings and Elion's drugs prompted the formation of a strong coordinated research effort directed against acute leukemia. In the mid-1950s a powerful group of young scientists was assembled by Dr. C. Gordon Zubrod at the National Cancer Institute (NCI) in Bethesda, Maryland, to bring chemistry, pharmacology, and quantitative clinical trials all to bear on this one disease. The major players at NCI were two unusual young men with confusingly similar names. One was Emil Frei III—known as Tom. The other was Emil J Freireich—known as J (no period after the J).

Like their boss, Zubrod, and unlike the vast majority of their teachers and peers, Tom and J were convinced that leukemia could be cured, if only enough smart minds and money could be applied to the problem. Capitalizing on the unprecedented human and financial resources available at NCI, Frei and Freireich concentrated on understanding the clinical manifestations of childhood leukemia and finding new treatments for its deadly twin complications of infection and bleeding. Instead of dying quickly from these dreaded complications, the sick children would survive long enough for the new drugs to have time to be tested. This was absolutely critical for other treatments to have any chance of success. Frei and Freireich and their younger associates discovered that, when a child relapsed from leukemia, the new growth often first showed up in the brain rather than in the bone marrow; they formulated a whole new strategy to prevent this from happening.

Gordon Zubrod, Tom, and J also saw the need for new methods of comparing the results of one study with another. How else could they know whether they had improved the odds of remission or life expectancy? For the first time they defined quantitatively what it meant to be "in remission," and they systematically compared the effectiveness of new agents against the old. It sounds like a simple task to define and quantitate the status of a patient at any given time, but it was then an unprecedented approach.

Yet their boldest stroke was to combine a number of potent drugs into a single treatment. They reasoned that, while each drug had antileukemic effects, each also had *different* side effects against normal tissues. Thus the antileukemic effects could be cumulative, whereas the toxicity would not be. Zubrod and his associates tried this approach even though it ran counter to the powerful voices of some of the more established experts—controversy over their treatment became particularly tense when they sought to obtain large quantities of precious blood platelets to transfuse into children who were bleeding to death. Ethical issues never before addressed in medicine emerged at every turn, humanitarian dilemmas confronting scientific opportunities for the first time in medical history.

The Leukemia Service at the NCI during the 1950s was an exciting place to be. The many young doctors who, like myself, spent one or two years on the service as part of their military obligation (Public Health Service) brought a steady stream of energetic and talented people into contact with their young laboratory chiefs, who were game to try anything within reason. It is not an exaggeration to point out that many of those who trained at the NIH became the leaders of medical research throughout the United States in the second half of the century.

Zubrod, Frei, and Freireich at NCI unquestionably formed the hub of leukemia research, but they readily admit that key pieces were contributed by scientists on, as it were, the periphery. Three scientists did work that proved especially noteworthy, and their stories round off the epic of leukemia research. Howard Skipper, Ph.D., at the Kettering Institute in Birmingham, Alabama, in the 1950s and early 1960s showed how to cure experimental leukemia in mice, giving researchers an alternative to clinical trials for new drugs and treatments. Dr. James Holland, who started the Leukemia Service at NCI and soon moved to Roswell Park Memorial Cancer Institute in Buffalo, New York, oversaw the collaboration between the NCI scientists and an enormous number of investigators at hospitals all over the United States and some abroad. Holland's coordination made it possible to keep track of the results for a very large number of children with leukemia and to document a steady record of improved survival in successive studies. And finally, we return to Dr. Donald Pinkel. After his early training and work with Sidney Farber, Pinkel went on to St. Jude Children's Research Hospital in Memphis, Tennessee, to develop an aggressive treatment against the recurrence of leukemia in the brain and spinal cord (as well as bone marrow), an essential part of eradicating all leukemia cells in the body following the use of combination chemotherapy.

Pinkel's career serves to frame the history of the cure of childhood leukemia presented here. He was there as a junior scientist in the first days of groping, those hesitant, intuitive, small-scale, desperate attempts to find some foothold on a cliff no one else thought could be scaled in a lifetime. And he was there at the summit, making the last bold yet deliberate effort that brought the prize within grasp. His clinical studies capped the creative achievements of the rest and finally made it possible to cure more than half of the children with leukemia. When he began, there was no hope of saving the life of a child with leukemia. When he finished, hope, not despair, prevailed.

Although each chapter describes the work of one scientist, the lines between their work become tangled—often productively. Along the way there were sometimes more failures than successes, as some lines ended in a blind alley. The cost of failure was the same as the value of each success, that of a child's life. But before a certain point, there was never any permanent success, and after a certain point, it became the norm.

PART II

The
Pioneers

CHAPTER 3

Donald Pinkel, M.D.: Beginnings

For every man the world is as fresh as it was at the first day, and as full of novelties for him who has the eyes to see them.

—Thomas Henry Huxley

"I became interested in children with leukemia at the very beginning of my medical career when I was just a second-year medical student at the University of Buffalo Medical School in 1949. I chose Hematology, the study of blood, as an elective course. This was taught at the County Hospital of Buffalo, where I could make rounds with three or four very busy hematologists and see all of their patients. It so happened that one of the first patients I saw was a child who had acute lymphocytic leukemia.

"A new drug called aminopterin had just been reported as being active in treating acute lymphocytic leukemia, but the hematologists at that hospital felt the drug was too toxic to use, that it had too many side effects. They actually gave me an ampule of aminopterin to try in experiments on rats, but they refused to treat the child with that same drug. It was not for lack of caring. They simply believed that acute lymphocytic leukemia was universally fatal and that the hematologist's job was over as soon as the diagnosis was made. The hematologist would turn the child back to the pediatrician, whose job it was to explain to the family that the child was going to die. They might give blood transfusions to extend the life of the child for a few days or weeks and to give the family time to absorb the shock of the diagnosis, but that was truly the state of affairs at that time.

"Then, in my first week as an intern at the Children's Hospital in Buffalo in 1951, one of my first patients was a child, about three years old, who was bleeding in the skin and from the nose and who had a fever, infection, and anemia: I made the diagnosis of acute lymphocytic leukemia. The philosophy about the disease, and indeed the reality, was that this child was going to die in the near future. It was a traumatic event for me as a new intern to be responsible for a patient who had a fatal disease, especially in a field like pediatrics where you expect that your patients will get better.

"To prepare myself for the difficult task of telling the family the bad news, I first went to a child psychiatrist and we sat down and talked together. This child had no private physician: he was what we used to call a ward case on the public service, and the intern was the doctor responsible for such patients. The family, of course, found it very difficult to accept the diagnosis, and they were quite distraught. We had just started using cortisone at that time, so this child received cortisone as well as methotrexate, the standard treatment in 1951. You see, by then, pediatrics had evolved to the point that we were at least treating patients with acute leukemia—in adults this was not nearly so standard. But we used cortisone and methotrexate together and were able to induce a clinical remission in about 50 percent of the children. We were able to send them home looking well, feeling well, and often able to go back to school temporarily. That was a big step forward.

"This particular child did develop a remission but it lasted for only about three or four months. When this child and other comparable children developed active leukemia once again, we again tried the cortisone and methotrexate. When that wouldn't work, we'd use ACTH [*adrenocortico-tropin hormone*—the pituitary-derived hormone that stimulates the adrenal glands] and sometimes we would get a temporary improvement from that. But most children were dead in six months to a year even though they had temporary improvement.

"When the other interns and the senior physicians and nurses discovered that I had a special interest in children's leukemia, I think some were horrified, regarding this as some type of ghoulish fascination. Back then, when we made rounds, if we found that a patient on the ward had leukemia or any other form of advanced cancer, when we got to that room someone would say 'leukemia' and there would be no further discussion. We'd pass by the door and go on to the next patient. The thing that impressed upon me and concerned me more than anything else was the sense of hopelessness in the minds of physicians and other professionals in regard to these children. It troubled me deeply that they were not receiving attention. It was not that people didn't care, but rather that the care-givers couldn't handle that situation. It didn't take long for the nurses to discover that, if they had a child with leukemia on their service, when none of the doctors wanted to go and talk with the family or do a physical examination or give a blood transfusion or prescribe narcotics, I would do it, even though I wasn't stationed on that ward. I had no objection to using narcotics or sedatives, and I was quite willing to prescribe drugs to relieve the anxiety, pain, and discomfort of children. And, if I can say so myself, I was a pretty good technician. That was important, because doing procedures on children is difficult and the child appreciates skill with needles and with other procedures. I remember the gratitude of the families when I would help the children through the tough times.

"We really did try to keep the blood tests and bone marrow studies to a minimum in order not to traumatize the patients unnecessarily. That was important to the children and to their parents. The main procedure at the time was giving whole blood transfusions to replace the blood they would hemorrhage: sometimes we were fortunate enough to have fresh blood rather than the older bank blood, but packed red blood cell transfusions and platelet packs to actually prevent the bleeding were not yet available. But if I had done nothing else but give the child and the family the sense that they were cared about and being cared for, then that in itself was perhaps a worthwhile contribution.

"Seeing the children go into remission was the exciting, memorable part of those early experiences for me. I would drop into the hematology clinic and see them when they came back for their outpatient visits. I became more and more involved with these children. So, when I became a chief resident in my third year, I was offered the opportunity to set up a tumor registry and a tumor clinic, for children with leukemia and other forms of childhood cancer.

"Support from the Erie County Unit of the American Cancer Society allowed us to employ a part-time secretary and tumor registrar. We began to have regular multidisciplinary meetings to evaluate children with leukemia and other types of cancer. This was probably one of the first pediatric tumor board conferences anywhere, and it was an important step in improving the quality of medical care for children with cancer.

"I would examine all of the children who had cancer even though I was only chief resident, because I was functioning at the level of an attending physician as far as these children were concerned. In fact, when I completed my year as chief resident, my cancer duties were turned over to a full professor. That was a formative year for me: it helped me to decide that I would dedicate my life to working with children who had cancer.

"I applied for a fellowship to support my further training at Memorial Sloan-Kettering in New York. It was unusual at that time for a pediatrician to make a specialty of childhood cancer. A cancer surgeon named Glenn Leak who was a Memorial graduate, coordinator of cancer education for the medical school, and a leader in the American Cancer Society, used to come over to the Children's Hospital and encourage me by saying, 'We need somebody to take care of these children with cancer.' On the other hand, the pediatric faculty was skeptical, telling me in so many words, 'You're throwing away your career.' The prevailing attitude was that cancer was not a big pediatric problem and even if it were, there was nothing we could do about it anyway. But, being in charge of the tumor program, I found out that, in children over the age of one at Children's Hospital, cancer was the leading cause of death: the figures proved that cancer *was* a major childhood problem.

"In the early 1950s there was interesting work going on at Memorial with 6-mercaptopurine [6-MP], the work of Joe Burchenal and Dave Karnofsky [see Chapter 4]. The drug became available for our own patients just as soon as it was found to be useful in leukemia in 1952. We used it right away and there was much excitement in the air because we now had three drugs that were active; 6-MP, methotrexate, and prednisone. Particularly exciting was the fact that 6-mercaptopurine was a specifically designed chemical inhibitor. It wasn't just luck that it was found. I was very impressed with the thinking of Hitchings and Elion who had logically designed a compound to do a particular job in inhibiting cancer cells [see Chapters 5 and 6]. If we could sit down and think about the metabolism of cancer cells and use the new information about DNA structure, we could come up with agents that would interfere with the vital processes of the leukemia cell and then, perhaps, we'd be able to go all the way. So there was a great sense of optimism."

Events prevented Dr. Pinkel from taking his fellowship training at Memorial. A few weeks before he was scheduled to start, he was ordered to active duty in the army reserve as the head of the Pediatrics Service in the hospital at Fort Devens, Massachusetts. There he became very ill with severe poliomyelitis and ended up as a patient himself in an army hospital. After six months in the hospital, he was transferred to the Veterans Administration Hospital in West Roxbury, outside Boston. During his recovery, Don had to learn how to drive a car again. The first day he had a license, he drove to Boston Children's Hospital and met the famous Dr. Sidney Farber, who also had strong ties to Buffalo. (Pinkel's former chief in Buffalo was a friend of Dr. Farber's.) Farber offered Pinkel a position as a research fellow at the Children's Cancer Research Foundation, then called 'the Jimmy Fund Clinic. So Pinkel's work in the clinic became part of his polio rehabilitation.

"I had much weakness in my legs in those days, which I still have, but at that time I was still wearing long leg braces and using crutches. Gradually I reduced my dependency to the point of only using short leg braces and a cane. I was coming along well, getting daily rehabilitation treatments at the Veterans Hospital and then working a full day at the Jimmy Fund Clinic. *Advances in Cancer Research* had asked Dr. Farber to write a review article on human cancer chemotherapy for its 1956 volume, and he asked me to work on it for him. I reviewed all the world literature on cancer chemotherapy—which was possible for one person to do at that time. Imagine what that task would be like today! This grounded me firmly in what was happening in the whole field of chemotherapy.

"That year, 1956, besides seeing many patients, doing many procedures, and prescribing a great deal of steroids, methotrexate, and 6-MP, I really did two things. I was given a new drug, actinomycin-D, to evaluate. I did the initial evaluation and described the dosage and toxicity of the drug in patients and its effectiveness in certain types of children's cancer, Wilms' tumor [a kidney tumor] and rhabdomyosarcoma [a cancer originating in embryonic muscle]. Actinomycin-D was a very important drug in many ways. It was the first antibiotic—that is, it was derived from bacterial sources—that showed a useful effect in shrinking human cancer: specifically, it was the first drug of any kind to destroy Wilms' tumor and rhabdomyosarcoma. Biologically, it was interesting because it had a different means of killing cancer cells from the other drugs that we had, and that was exciting as well. It was particularly gratifying to see the new agent cause disappearance of cancer once it had spread even to the lungs."

Why did someone like Pinkel, an investigator interested in childhood leukemia, begin to study other childhood cancers? First of all, if you specialize in children with cancer, you have to treat them all. These diseases are not so common that a doctor can specialize in only one form of cancer. Also, because there were then no effective drugs for these other cancers, it was best to try out new experimental drugs first on patients with no other hope of treatment. Finally, although actinomycin-D had been predicted from animal tests to be very effective in human leukemia, it turned out not to be very effective at all. It would reduce the white blood count, but it would not produce remissions. Consequently this drug was being tested in children who had forms of advanced cancer that were beyond any conventional therapy.

"Our first response in a child who had Wilms' tumor was in a youngster from Vermont—a French Canadian boy who had Wilms' tumor that had spread throughout his lungs. He was dying. I still remember injecting actinomycin-D. I had to use the vein on the back of his hand because we couldn't find any other veins; he'd had so many blood tests and intravenous treatments in the past. Back in those days, of course, we doctors did everything ourselves and we didn't have specially trained I.V. teams and chemotherapy nurses to start our intravenous treatments. After the initial treatment we sent the boy home; when he came back to the clinic I had a repeat x-ray made of his chest. When the x-ray was returned to me, the chest x-ray was normal. There was no sign of any tumor in the lungs. I assumed that they had mixed up the x-rays with another patient, so I sent him down to get another x-ray of the chest. I got an angry call from the radiologist: 'What do you think you're doing sending this child down for another x-ray? You just ordered one on him a short time ago!' And I said, 'I think his must have been mixed up with someone else's x-ray because the lungs on this x-ray are clear.' He retorted, 'You dummy, don't you know a response when you get one?'

"Then we had another child who was dying of sarcoma of the back of the throat that was blocking passage of food and air. This child also had a good tumor regression. Unfortunately the improvements in both of these children were only temporary, but Dr. Farber was enthused and decided that we should start using actinomycin-D in patients with Wilms' tumor after their initial surgery. This was the beginning of what is now called adjuvant chemotherapy. His idea was that, if one took out most of the tumor with surgery and were left with only minimal disease, one had a better chance of curing it than if one were treating the whole tumor in the first place—especially when the patient had a large tumor. So we began to use actinomycin-D as an adjuvant following surgery, and that principle, surgery followed by chemotherapy, is still widely used today."

"As the year wound down the opportunity arose for me to go back to Buffalo, to Roswell Park Memorial Cancer Institute. Its director, Dr. George Moore, had been given a large budget by the state health commissioner of New York to make this into a research institute as well as a treatment center. When I had been chief resident in Buffalo before my Boston experience, I had gone over to meet George Moore soon after he had arrived. I told him that I was interested in children with cancer and in making cancer research my career.

"At that time he indicated the possibility of starting a pediatric unit at Roswell Park. While I was working for Dr. Farber, George checked around on my references and then asked me to return to Buffalo to begin the new pediatric unit there. Unfortunately Roswell Park did not have the specialized service departments—x-ray, clinical laboratories, blood bank, nursing care, and all of the other things that make up a successful pediatric program. In April 1956 I was given space on 5 East, which at that time was being used for storage, and told to start a pediatric unit there, both for pediatric care and for research. There was a lot of work to do simply to get nurses who could take care of children, to establish policies and practices that were conducive to good child care, let alone to deliver specialized care to children with cancer.

"That was exciting! I was only twenty-nine years old. I had the advantage of being from Buffalo—it's my home, it's where I was trained, and I had many friends and knew all of the pediatricians. I could get referrals of patients to my service because all the doctors were aware of my interest in children who had cancer and leukemia. Many of them thought I was crazy and they frankly told me so. 'All of those kids dying of cancer over there, how do you do it?' Everyone said that if you valued your career as a doctor, you had to specialize in something that offered more possibility of success.

"I was the only pediatrician at Roswell Park—I was it. It was tough, demanding work all of the time. I had the highest mortality rate of any pediatrician in the area and it was often discouraging. When you are losing children, it's difficult to believe that you're making any headway in terms of a cure. True, we were achieving remissions in many of our children and we were finding new drugs like cyclophosphamide (Cytoxan) and vincristine that would produce remissions. But we weren't reducing the mortality, that is, the children would have temporary remissions and then they would relapse and die. There were many times when I left that ward in the evening and didn't know how I was going to return to work again the next day. It could be devastating at times and I couldn't really discuss it with anyone, not even my wife. I knew that no one else could quite understand what I was going through. It's like a lot of bad experiences that people have. You can't explain it to other people, they don't understand what's wrong with you.

"Yet I knew that at any time I could walk out of there, leave leukemia behind, set out my shingle in private pediatric practice and double my income. (When I went to Roswell Park I started out with a salary of $9,000 a year, part of which came from research funds provided by the philanthropist Mary Lasker. I told George that $9,000 was the minimum required to support my wife and four children. After a year or so, I was making a salary of $14,000, gigantic back in 1957.)

"I had my own children to go home to and play with and enjoy, no matter how bad things got at the hospital. I like music and I like to swim. But the main thing that kept me going was the courage of the children who were my patients. I'd say to myself, 'If these children can face cancer and their parents can face it every day, then what's wrong with me?' I remember so clearly that strong feeling. Another strong motivating feeling was that, if I don't take care of them, who will? Just as when I was an intern, I thought that, even if I'm not doing them any good medically— which indeed a lot of people thought—if I only give the family and the children the feeling that society and the community are concerned about them, and want to help them, then that's important.

"It was a continuous struggle to maintain an active growing medical unit where one could do research and organize the kind of patient care that was needed. Hospital administrators tended to look down on pediatric oncology, no doubt wondering what was the point of spending all that time with these parents and children when all of these children were dying anyway. So we had to keep fighting to obtain and retain the resources to run the pediatric unit and to justify adequate clinic space, or nursing help, or social service help, or play therapists. Administrators and doctors who only treat adults often don't realize how important these can be to the care of sick children."

In the five and a half years that Don Pinkel spent at Roswell Park, his average working day was twelve hours long, six and a half days a week. At the same time that he had so much responsibility for building up the pediatrics unit, he was doing research in the laboratory, analyzing data, and publishing papers.

Roswell Park was a congenial place for a young medical researcher. "It was growing very fast as an institution, but it was small enough that you could get hold of it. There were lots of good, active scientists and clinicians, and they were very supportive and permitted me to innovate. Dr. Moore pretty much left me alone—that was his style. He gave someone a job, and he was off doing his own thing (he was an expert on growing human cancer cells in tissue culture).

"In pediatrics, leukemia was our main interest. The chief of medicine, Jim Holland, was handling the Adult Acute Leukemia Service. He had teamed up with Tom Frei and J Freireich at the National Cancer Institute for a cooperative group study of leukemia, so I joined their group. We used to meet in Washington every six weeks at the National Institutes of Health conference center to discuss the first comparative studies of leukemia treatment.

"I saw an increasing number of children who went into remission with the drugs we were using, but who developed leukemic cells in the lining [meninges] of the brain and spinal cord before relapsing with leukemia in the bone marrow. Actually, I'd been aware of this when I was working with Dr. Farber in Boston: there we began using methotrexate injected into the spinal fluid as a way to relieve the symptoms associated with leukemia cells in the spinal fluid such as severe headaches, seizures, and paralysis of cranial nerves.

"At Roswell Park I learned that there was a relationship between the duration of a leukemia remission and the risk of relapse taking place in the central nervous system (CNS). The longer the remission, the greater the chance that, when relapse occurred, it would be in the CNS. Short remissions usually ended with relapse in the bone marrow instead. Jim Holland and I talked a lot about this, and we talked about the possibility of radiating the meninges to try to prevent the children from getting CNS relapse. We also talked about possibly injecting methotrexate into the CNS before the CNS got involved with leukemia."

With Holland and Walter Murphy, chief of the Department of Radiation Therapy, Pinkel began his first experiments with radiation of the brain. The doses were very small, too small to make a difference. But the idea kept fermenting.

In 1961 Don Pinkel became the first director of St. Jude Children's Research Hospital in Memphis, Tennessee. There he had an opportunity to create a new kind of pediatrics institution and to pursue the leukemia research he had first mulled over in Buffalo. Both the hospital and his research there had phenomenal results, but that part of the story will come later. First, we must turn back to the other scientists whose intertwining strands of research had brought about the striking progress Pinkel had witnessed in a little more than a decade after his first despairing encounter with a leukemic child in 1949.

CHAPTER 4

Joseph Burchenal, M.D.

Keep on going and the chances are you will stumble on something, perhaps when you are least expecting it. I have never heard of anyone stumbling on something sitting down.
—Charles Kettering

Joseph Burchenal, unlike most of the medical researchers we will meet in this book, knew early on that he wanted to be a scientist. In 1920, when he was an eight-year-old in Wilmington, Delaware, he was captivated by his cousin's chemistry set and soon acquired one of his own. Together the cousins tried to make gunpowder from flour, sulfur, crude saltpeter, and homemade charcoal. The flashes were spectacular and satisfying, and it was sheer luck they did not blow themselves up. Joe's love affair with chemistry began in those happy days puttering around with his Chemcraft set.

Another relative pointed his interest toward chemotherapy: his great-uncle John, a general practitioner, was an enthusiastic prescriber of quinine. Malaria, he'd say, was a very bad disease, and if quinine was strong enough to cure the malaria, it would probably cure anything else that ailed you, including the common cold and stomachache. As a result, all the Burchenal children were dosed with Uncle John's "Magnificent Capsules"—a powerful concoction of quinine, podophyllin (a purgative extracted from May-apples, derivatives of which are, curiously, now used in cancer chemotherapy), and various other natural products. Taking this powerful medicine—the usual prescription was for three days' worth—made the sick child feel much worse. Whether or not the Magnificent Capsules helped the underlying illness, Joe always felt practically cured once the medicine was stopped. The memory of that family remedy lingered with him as he did his own research into chemical treatments.

Joe's interest in chemistry was stimulated further by good teachers at

Exeter Academy, and again at Princeton University, where his premedical program was heavily laced with chemistry courses.

His plan to become a doctor was spurred in part by his lawyer-father's conviction that everyone should leave the world a better place and that the best way to do so was to practice a profession. But far more important was a family tragedy. During Joe's freshman year at Princeton, his mother had her leg amputated for bone cancer (osteogenic sarcoma). The surgeon, a professor at the University of Pennsylvania's medical school, explained that he thought that the operation had removed all of her cancer; however, if it were to recur, it would likely spread to her lungs and then nothing could be done. Sadly, two years later, the disease recurred in her lungs, and Joe's mother died of cancer.

Joe now faced a difficult decision. He had finished his premedical requirements at Princeton and had applied to several medical schools near Philadelphia. But should he go? He still had a nine-year-old sister at home, the year was 1933, the depths of the Depression, and his family was barely solvent. The low medical school tuition—only five hundred dollars a year—at the University of Pennsylvania persuaded him to stick to his goal of becoming a medical scientist. He wanted, in a vague, unformed way, to learn more about cancer, to find a chemical treatment that would control the disease once it had spread beyond the reach of a surgeon's knife, as it had with his mother.

In his naiveté and youth, he had no idea that the experts of the day thought the task impossible. Even chemotherapy for bacterial infections was considered hopeless. When Joe asked a bacteriology lab instructor about the possibility of curing bloodstream infections, he was told the chances were essentially nil. When, for example, mercurochrome, that excellent antiseptic sterilizer for the skin, had been tried intravenously against streptococcus infection, it proved impossible to cure the infection without killing the patient.

For all the skepticism of teachers and experts, Joe continued to be fascinated by the chemical treatment of cancer. He kept reading the medical literature on the treatment of animal tumors, and the summer after his sophomore year in medical school, he actually set up a small laboratory to do studies on fifty white rats. From Columbia University he got a rat bearing the Jensen sarcoma, a kind of cancer that can be transplanted from one rat into many other rats. He removed a part of the original rat's tumor and sliced the cancerous tissue into tiny pieces, injected the bits of tissue into the fifty rats, and waited for the tumors to appear. The plan was to treat the rats with insulin, which at that time was thought to have some effect in inhibiting animal tumors. But the intended experiment never really got under way because, as he was surprised to find, the tumors in the rats grew to very different sizes, even before the insulin treatment. There was no way to measure the results of treatment without a standardized system, and the technique of standardizing and quantitating the growth of tumors had not yet been developed. Without a reproducible system, there was no way to know if the drug was working—unless all of the tumors disappeared, which they didn't. Thus "my very first experiment with cancer came to naught, as would so many others in future years."

Joe was aware that ten years earlier, in the mid-1920s, the son of President Calvin Coolidge had developed a tennis blister and died of streptococcus blood poisoning. Then, while at medical school, a colleague of Joe's accidentally stuck herself with a needle that contained streptococci, and she was ill for many months. Antibiotics were not available then, but by the end of Joe's time in medical school, he did witness a very elaborate apparatus for injecting the red dye Prontosil into the spinal fluid in order to treat meningitis.

Joe spent a two-month stretch at the Pediatric Service of Baltimore's Union Memorial Hospital where he saw patients with childhood leukemia and, thanks to an outstanding hematologist, Dr. Walter Baetjer, was able to spend an hour or two each evening reviewing the blood slides of those patients and learning the mysteries of white blood cells as they could be studied under the microscope. Like many other physicians, Joe was staggered to see how very aggressive leukemia was, how rapidly it progressed, and how much, in that respect at least, it resembled a severe and overwhelming bacterial infection. Had Joe gone to medical school just a few years earlier, making that comparison between leukemia and infection would not have suggested a new line of cancer research. But while Joe was going through his medical training, sulfa drugs were just becoming established as antibiotics. By the time he graduated, sulfa drugs were the standard treatment against streptococcal infections and were finding uses against the most common and deadly form of pneumonia as well. (For many older doctors today, the advent of potent antibiotics has been the most striking change in medical treatment of their lifetime.) Joe reasoned that if infectious diseases—the biggest killers of all—could be defeated by chemistry, why not cancer? And why not start with the cancer that was most like a fast, deadly infection: acute leukemia in children? This fortunate decision guided the rest of his scientific career. Determined to specialize in childhood cancer, the young Dr. Burchenal took further postgraduate training at New York Hospital.

In the late 1930s, the interns and residents ate together with the faculty in a beautiful paneled dining room on the eighteenth floor of the hospital. There Joe first met Dr. Jacob Furth, an outstanding experimentalist and leading authority on leukemia in mice. During his illustrious career, this very gentle scientist, with his extraordinary knowledge of the scientific literature and his provocative questions (always delivered with heavy Germanic expression in a high-pitched voice), inspired a great many young doctors. Dr. Furth offered Joe the opportunity of working in his laboratory on off-duty nights and of pursuing a research project as well: the relationship of pregnancy to leukemia in mice. Furth had previously found that he could transplant leukemic cells into genetically susceptible mice, even with a single leukemic cell, and he suggested that Joe study whether leukemic cells in pregnant mice would penetrate the placenta and transfer leukemia from mother to the "pups," as baby mice are called.

Joe learned to inoculate leukemic cells into a particular strain (AK) of female mice: the mice developed leukemia before they were fertilized. He also inoculated females with leukemic cells during the course of their pregnancy. In both instances, the females became very sick with their leukemia at about the time of their delivery, but the outcome of the experiments was always the same—the pups were born healthy and without the disease, despite the advanced leukemic condition of the mothers.

The pups were foster-nursed by nonleukemic mice for a few days, and then they were carefully observed for periods of up to three months. This was well beyond the time when an adult mouse injected with even a single cell of leukemia would be expected to live, and yet the pups never developed any evidence of leukemia. Furthermore, Joe's survey of the literature showed that children who were born to leukemic mothers did not have leukemia either.

By contrast, the infants of mothers who had viral infections were born infected with the same viral disease as their mothers. This series of experiments in mice seemed to demonstrate that the passage of leukemic cells was different from the passage of virus infection. On the basis of the experimental data, Joe and his teacher concluded that mouse leukemia was not transmitted by a virus.

They were wrong, however. "We came to the erroneous conclusion about the nature of this type of mouse leukemia, erroneous because we weren't as smart as Dr. Ludwig Gross, who later showed that the leukemia virus *was* transmitted through the placenta, but one simply had to wait a longer period of time in order to see the expression of leukemia."

Burchenal wasn't the only one to fail with this approach, of course. Even after Gross published his remarkable finding—that leukemia could be produced in pups of leukemic mothers if the conditions were "right"—many investigators still had trouble reproducing the very tricky experiments. Yet Gross did show that mouse leukemia was due to a virus. The relevance of that to human leukemia is still not clear.

At New York Hospital Joe also met Dr. Claude Forkner, a famous hematologist who had recently completed a great comprehensive tome on leukemia. His office was very close to the pediatric floor, so late in the evening Joe would bring in blood slides from his leukemic patients for help in interpreting them. Dr. Forkner, like Dr. Baetjer, always seemed to find time to instruct the young doctor in white cell morphology. It was he who suggested that anyone interested in hematology should go to the Thorndike Laboratory at Boston City Hospital, which was part of the Harvard Medical Service. The research there was directed by Dr. George Minot and Dr. William Castle, who had been instrumental in discovering the nature and cure of pernicious anemia, a monumental discovery in its own right.

The move to Boston was postponed to let Joe go to Europe and work in several laboratories. He also intended the trip to serve as a sort of honeymoon for himself and his new bride, Margaret Pembroke Thom ("Tommy"). The naive young newlyweds set out for France in 1939. Their timing was very poor. Paris was full of soldiers, and the German laboratories had to be ruled out. They went to Switzerland instead. Then one day while they were hiking over the mountain passes between Lucerne and Geneva, war broke out in Europe and all of their plans again had to be changed. Joe and Tommy stayed in Switzerland, allowing Joe to work at the Zurich Kinderspital under the famous Dr. Fanconi on children's tumors and leukemias, and at the Universitätsklinik learning to interpret slides from the new bone marrow aspiration technique under Dr. Karl Rohr.

In December Joe received a letter from Dr. Minot in Boston, indicating that he had a "half of a half-salary" available for a fellowship position beginning in January. Minot, a very frugal man, knew that there were many more people who wanted to work with him than he could accommodate. His hospital allotted him six salaries for medical fellows, but he divided the salaries in half in order to take on twelve fellows. One of these fellows was due to leave by the end of December, and Minot prepared to play the game again. He divided that salary in half to gain two more fellows and that was the "half" offered to Joe. Joe knew that, if he accepted the meager offer, there was no guarantee that he would be kept on beyond June. But full of the confidence of youth, he and his wife took a boat from Italy back home.

When Dr. Burchenal joined the Harvard group in January of 1940, he was assigned to work on a disease called polycythemia vera. This disease is characterized by the production of excessive amounts of blood. The combination of high blood pressure and sluggish flow of blood due to its high viscosity puts the patients in danger of having a myocardial infarction or a stroke. Joe and his colleagues had to obtain bone marrow samples from normal people as well as from patients with polycythemia vera. They needed to obtain enough bone marrow to measure the extent to which it was saturated with oxygen: a task that, in turn, used extremely elaborate apparatus. Starting from the observation that low oxygen concentration stimulates red cell production (notably in people who live at high altitudes), the Harvard group was trying to find out whether the bone marrow was being stimulated to produce more blood cells because it was low in oxygenation.

Before anything else could be studied, the Harvard group had to find a way to sample the bone marrow. In itself this was a fairly new procedure. Joe made his own needles for this purpose by adapting needles that were used to do spinal taps. The first bone marrow samples had to be taken from normal subjects.

Joe taught another of the fellows, Dr. C. P. Emerson, how to do sternal puncture, and his first subject was the principal investigator, Dr. Joseph Burchenal himself. It was a bit painful, Joe recalled, and hard to locate the exact source of the pain. He couldn't tell whether it was coming from his breastbone, where the needle had been placed, or from the back. (The pressure of withdrawing marrow causes pain locally in the bone and also pain that is "referred" to the back.)

While working with this group of hematologists Joe again learned a great deal about experimental methodology. Dr. Castle was studying the effects of different vitamin B_{12} substances on pernicious anemia and also the effects of normal gastric juice, essential for the intestinal absorption of vitamin B_{12}, which is notably absent in patients with pernicious anemia. Because patients lack the so-called intrinsic factor in gastric juice, they cannot absorb the normal amount of vitamin B_{12} from their diet. The scientists added different types of food extracts to the diet of the patients to see if these would correct the defect, measuring this by a rise in blood counts. If the counts didn't improve in their patients, then as a control, they would try to improve them with a ten-day course of feeding dried hog stomach, which does contain the intrinsic factor. The idea was that if the substance they were testing didn't improve the blood count and the hog stomach material did, then they knew that the experimental mixture was not effective in correcting the defect of pernicious anemia.

The study of patients with this disease afforded an ideal situation in which to do that kind of experiment, because the patients were not so ill that a negative experiment for ten days would in any way compromise their condition. Joe was to find out later how much more difficult it was to study new drugs in patients with acute leukemia, but for now, learning this experimental methodology served him well.

Joe was struck by a patient he saw as he made rounds with Henry Jackson, another famous hematologist. This woman's acute leukemia went into remission after she had fought off a bout of pneumonia, which her doctors had successfully treated with sulfadiazine: they also treated the patient with liver extract. The doctors weren't aware at that time that, very occasionally, spontaneous remission in leukemia sometimes occurs after resolution of a severe infection. There was a great deal of excitement after the patient improved and went home, and Joe visited her there every two weeks to take her blood counts. Her remission lasted for nine months. When she did relapse, he gave her the same treatment—minus the pneumonia, of course—but this did not produce a second remission and the patient died.

World War II forced Dr. Burchenal to turn away from his study of cancer chemotherapy. As a doctor in the military, his primary duty was the care of soldiers with infectious diseases. He had taken a reserve commission with the Fifth General Hospital, the "Harvard Unit," half a year before

Pearl Harbor. A month after the United States entered the war, his group was sent to northern Ireland, where they set up a hospital at the same time that the First Armored Division came into Glasgow, with about half of the soldiers very ill with yellow jaundice. His ward had eighty men sick with hepatitis B, caused by contaminated human serum that had been used in preparing the yellow fever vaccine that they had all received a few weeks before leaving the States. Fortunately, none died.

When the hospital moved to Salisbury, England, Joe's assignment as chief of infectious diseases meant preparing for the epidemics of meningitis, diphtheria, and other infectious diseases that were expected to result from the overcrowded conditions in the London Underground, then being used as a shelter during the bombing raids of London. These epidemics never did occur, but there were plenty of other infectious disease to make the job interesting and hectic. These experiences would serve him well years later in caring for children with leukemia, who often died of infectious diseases.

Right after D-Day, the Fifth General Hospital was ordered to Normandy. Joe set up an infectious disease ward made up entirely of tents arranged in checkerboard fashion in order to isolate different diseases in each separate tent. From there they moved on to establish a forward position on the French frontier, and so it went during the war.

Personal tragedy brought Joe home on leave. His wife had died suddenly, and he wanted to make sure that their young daughter would be brought up in Wilmington, Delaware, in the family of close friends with children her own age until he was able to get back to civilian life. He was still in the States on VE-Day, and the army refused to let him rejoin his unit—by that time, the troops were headed the other way. In expectation of assignment to the South Pacific, Joe requested training in tropical diseases at the Walter Reed Army Institute of Tropical Medicine in Washington, D.C. During the superb three-month course, he celebrated VJ-Day.

The Surgeon General's office next appointed Joe chief of the Tropical Medicine section at the Walter Reed Army Hospital, also in Washington. Here he learned how to treat patients with all sorts of exotic tropical diseases and to try the newly developed antiparasitic drugs: chloroquine for malaria, stilbamidine antimony compounds for kala-azar, and other treatments for different types of parasites, worms, and dysentery illnesses. Joe reveled in his access to the resources of the Army Institute of Tropical Medicine and it was there that he first heard from another consultant in the Surgeon General's office of the very hush-hush work done during the war on chemical warfare compounds, the nitrogen mustards, which were said to be the most exciting lead available in the area of cancer research.

In December 1945, not long before Joe was due to be discharged from the service, a chance conversation with Dr. Hale Ham, chief of research for chemical warfare, gave Joe the chance to return to his first interest. Dr. Ham tried to hire him for his Chemical Warfare Unit but also happened to mention a new cancer research unit that his predecessor, Dr. C. P. Rhoads, was setting up at Memorial Sloan-Kettering in New York. Rhoads (inevitably known as "Dusty" to his colleagues) was extremely knowledgeable about pathology, hematology, and biochemistry as well as a superb speaker, fund-raiser, and scientific administrator. He was especially interested in having his new research staff test new chemical compounds against cancer. In particular, Rhoads was looking for someone to do research on both human leukemia and experimental leukemia in mice. This was exactly what Joe wanted to do. On March 8, 1946, he left the army and walked directly into Memorial Sloan-Kettering and the rest of his career.

Joe and his daughter moved to Connecticut. He bought a house and a third-hand Model A Ford to get to the train station, and arranged for a French governess to look after his child.

The new job brought personal as well as professional happiness. Among the bright Vassar graduates whom Dusty Rhoads had recruited to work as lab technicians was Joan Riley, whom Joe "eventually persuaded to take over the running of my life." They married in 1948. On New Year's morning, their new baby's crying alerted them to smoke; the family got out safely, but the house burned down. While walking through the woods soon after, Joe found a lovely piece of land, but the owner wanted $4,000. "I'm a poor starving medical fellow," he said, and heard in response, "I'm a poor starving widow of a clergyman." Sympathizing with each other's problems, the two struck a bargain. Joe and Joan built their dream house and have lived there since 1951. They have had seven children altogether.

Dusty Rhoads's ties to the Army Chemical Warfare Unit proved to be critical to the successes of the new cancer research group at Memorial Sloan-Kettering. Thanks to the military's access to the brightest young men and unlimited resources for research, the Chemical Warfare Unit at Edgewood Arsenal in Maryland was an ideal training ground for cancer pharmacologists. At Joe's initial interview with Rhoads, he met Dr. David

Karnofsky, temporarily assigned to Memorial from Edgewood Arsenal. The two became lifelong friends and colleagues. They made frequent trips to the arsenal, both to fetch nitrogen mustard compounds for testing on mice and patients with lymphoma and to confer with scientists there. Among those originally recruited by Rhoads to work on chemical weapons, Karnofsky, Howard Skipper, Fred Phillips, John Beasley, and Oscar Bodansky ended up making outstanding contributions to cancer research.

The hunt for chemical compounds that might be useful against cancer extended beyond the military to industry. The chief of experimental chemotherapy at Memorial, Dr. C. Chester Stock, set up agreements with pharmaceutical companies for his staff to study the usefulness of new compounds in experimental animals and in humans. Interesting compounds might have no obvious connection to biological processes: in 1948, for example, the Burchenal group found that an American Cyanamid compound intended to preshrink cotton, trimethylene melamine (TEM), turned out to keep leukemic mice alive longer than untreated mice. Joe's group found that TEM was very effective in temporarily "shrinking" cancerous lymph enlargements in patients with lymphoma, a malignancy also derived from lymphocytes.

The partial successes with TEM and nitrogen mustard compounds on mice and on patients with lymphoma and also chronic leukemia were both exciting and frustrating to Burchenal. Chemotherapy was helping some cancer patients. But for the patients he was most interested in, those with acute leukemia, the compounds they had tried so far were useless.

The frustration and hope were aroused still further with another new chemical: aminopterin. Joe had learned in 1947 that Dr. Sidney Farber of Boston Children's Hospital had been getting remissions with aminopterin in children with acute leukemia, and he eagerly accepted Farber's invitation to come see for himself. Joe was impressed by their results. Not only did the children's white blood counts fall and enlarged spleens and livers shrink, but their bone marrow returned to normal for a few months. Aminopterin's mode of action was striking as well. Its chemical structure closely resembled the newly discovered folic acid, but, rather than aiding metabolism as folic acid did, it deranged the metabolism of leukemic cells, very much in the way that sulfa drugs deranged the metabolism of bacterial cells.

With Farber's help, the Memorial group obtained some of the new antimetabolite from the brilliant Indian biochemist Dr. Subba Row at the

Lederle pharmaceutical company laboratories. The Lederle group was obsessed with the earlier successes at Mount Sinai and was determined to make derivatives of folic acid that could be used successfully to treat patients with cancer. But the researchers at Memorial initially saw no response at all. Rhoads and Karnofsky were dubious about the drug in any case, and the lack of positive results with the first nine children they treated with it only confirmed their skepticism. They were ready to write a paper for the medical journals proclaiming the drug to be ineffective, a paper they would have regretted later. But Joe told them to hold off: he could not forget his personal observations of the children under Farber's care. And then it happened: the tenth patient showed a good remission.

The contrast between the results of the Memorial group and the much better results of a group in Cincinnati under Dr. Guest—as many as six out of the seven of his patients treated with aminopterin had remissions—underscored the importance of having enough patients to detect uncommon events. These statistical variations in results were to be expected from any treatment that did not have a 100 percent success rate. In clinical research, a genuine response in a uniformly fatal disease, even though rare, can be a key lead in developing better treatments of the same general type. The fact that any remissions had occurred, even temporary ones, even in just a handful of patients, was important news to the world of chemotherapy.

Up to this point young Dr. Burchenal had prepared himself for a career in the research of childhood cancer, but had not made any original contributions. But now began a very rewarding relationship with Dr. George Hitchings, Gertrude Elion, and other scientists at the Burroughs Wellcome Company.

The experimental drugs to be used for acute leukemia in the next generation of studies were derivatives of normal purines, which are important components of nucleic acids, building blocks of the human system and particularly of DNA. The first of these chemical derivatives, 2,6-diaminopurine, was produced by George Hitchings around 1950, and it was a success: it shrank tumors and increased the survival time of leukemic mice. When Joe tested it in patients, he found that it produced partial remissions in cases of acute leukemia. The definition of remission had not yet been formalized; remission in this case simply meant that the blood counts improved. The counts did not revert completely to normal, however, and there continued to be signs of leukemia in the blood and bone marrow. Furthermore, the drug caused too much nausea and vomiting to be tolerated by most patients.

There was one spectacular result. The wife of a young clergyman experienced a complete remission for over two years. But then she relapsed, and the same drug did not work a second time. Clearly this did not seem to be a practical drug, but it was an important lead. The researchers were happily able to move on to a closely related but better drug, 6-mercaptopurine (6-MP), synthesized by Hitchings and Elion in 1951.

The new drug, 6-MP, roused the excitement of the entire program. First, Dr. Stock and Dr. Clarke at Memorial Sloan-Kettering Cancer Center found the drug to be very effective in mice who were bearing transplantable tumors. Next, Dr. Fred Phillips prepared the drug for experiments in patients by first studying its effects in dogs and showing how large a dose could be tolerated and what its side effects were. Most people can accept the use of mice in the testing process that is going to produce a possible cure for a serious disease. Far less acceptable is the necessity to upgrade the tests and learn more about effects by trying drugs on, for instance, dogs. Yet a drug that may possibly be useful to children, based on the work in mouse tumors, needs to have its toxicity evaluated in normal animals. Unfortunate as it may be, this is best done in dogs because they are generally similar to humans in the way they react to drugs. Joe Burchenal is not alone in saying that if it were not for animal studies, we would not have antileukemia drugs today. Through his involvement in this step-by-step process, Joe knew just what to look for in patients when he began to study it in the clinical situation.

There was another very important finding from the animal experiments. Researchers discovered, in mice, a type of cancer that was resistant to inhibition by folate analogs (aminopterin) and yet was still sensitive to being inhibited by 6-MP. This observation meant that, for the first time, there was an experimental way to study the problem of how to get around drug resistance. This was to assume even greater importance later, when there were additional drugs that could be used. (In one amusing episode that tells a lot about the early days of leukemia research, Joe put fifty mice that had been inoculated with leukemia cells into a cage which he wrapped in paper to take to Birmingham on an old DC-3 airplane. It was a particularly hot summer day and, once airborne, he took off the paper wrapping in order to let the mice breathe better. The smell was intense! Indeed, it was pungent, overwhelming, and sickening. The other passengers didn't thank the young scientist. Fortunately it was too late to put down again, or the pilot probably would have done so.) With the use of leukemic cells, the collaborating laboratory scientists were able to develop drug-resistant tumors so that they could study the effects of new drugs. They suspected that they would encounter similar problems in patients, and this is indeed what happened.

The Burchenal team was able to obtain temporary complete clinical and bone marrow–verified remissions in fifteen out of forty-five children with acute leukemia who were treated with 6-MP. They also found temporary improvement in some adults with acute leukemia. In keeping with the experiments in mice, some patients improved after treatment with 6-MP despite the fact that they had failed to respond to the folate antagonist, aminopterin. As with the mice, that particular observation was very encouraging, because it provided a handle on the problem of drug resistance. What defeats the chemotherapist is not that cells will not respond to treatment; indeed, it's possible to kill off 99.9 + percent of leukemic cells with a given drug. The problem is that the remaining few cells grow back, and when they do, they tend not to be responsive to a second course of treatment with the same drug.

In January 1953, Joe and his colleagues held an informal meeting at Memorial Sloan-Kettering for outstanding hematologists from around the world who were treating patients with acute leukemia. They offered to give out the compound 6-MP to investigators at other medical schools who wished to try it on patients who were resistant to standard methotrexate treatment. This effort led to ample confirmation in other centers.

To report the results at a major scientific meeting, Burchenal, Rhoads, and colleagues prepared an abstract to present to the American Society of Clinical Investigation—the "Young Turks" of academic medicine—at the annual clinical research meeting. That the abstract was not accepted for the program is indicative of the low esteem in which cancer chemotherapy was held at that time. It's hard to believe now that a major report of remissions of such a deadly disease by the use of a new drug would not have been considered of sufficient interest. The paper was presented instead, a short time later, at the annual meeting of the American Association for Cancer Research, probably a more suitable forum for this discovery in any event. Here it was greeted with great enthusiasm as an important advance.

While all this research was in progress, a common question that confronted Burchenal and his associates was whether patients should be told their diagnosis. In the 1940s and 1950s, and even into the 1960s, doctors generally did not tell their patients, particularly children, that they had cancer or leukemia. As we shall learn, however, it was subsequently discovered that patients are far more cooperative and satisfied with their medical care if they understand the issues.

For example, take the eleven-year-old girl with acute leukemia whom Dr. Burchenal treated in 1954 with 6-MP and another experimental drug. She went into a complete remission for eighteen months. But her disease relapsed nonetheless, and despite starting her back on the same medications, given in even higher doses, the marrow did not respond. At that point she was started on methotrexate, which by that time had replaced aminopterin as the most popular of the folate antagonists, and when she was treated with this drug, she went into a remission. The drug had troublesome side effects, particularly a sore mouth, and her dose was adjusted frequently in order to find just the right amount to control her disease without causing her too much toxicity. Eventually the program went well and the sores in her mouth disappeared.

Throughout all of this, the mother had remained insistent that the doctors not tell her daughter that she had leukemia. After the child had been in remission for a couple of years, however, a school friend told her, "You have leukemia and you're going to die." She responded, "I have leukemia but I'm not going to die!" The doctors had been concerned about what they would tell the child if she ever relapsed but, lo and behold, she never did. She may have been the first patient at Memorial to be truly cured of leukemia, although the doctors themselves could not believe that she had been cured at the time. She grew up, got married, and one day she came to the clinic and brought in a baby, an adopted child. When asked about this she said that her husband had been an adopted child, and he believed that adopted children were especially picked out by God. One lesson that we may draw from this lovely story is that, although parents often try to protect their children from knowing about their disease, patients have a way of finding out what's wrong with them, even though they may go along with the charade for a long time. It's often better to let them know and enlist their determination.

One of the more important influences on Joe's outlook on the chemotherapy of leukemia came early in 1963, when an oncologist who had previously been a fellow with them called from Baltimore to invite him to give the Mother Seton Memorial Lecture at St. Agnes Hospital in May. He suggested that the subject be "Long-Term Survivors in Children with Acute Leukemia." Joe agreed, supposing this to be a lecture in honor of a retiring Mother Superior of the hospital, and proceeded to put the matter aside for the moment. Imagine his surprise when about a month later *Life* magazine came out with a cover story on Mother Seton. Joe learned to his amazement that Mother Seton had been declared venerable by the Pope in 1957 and was about to be beatified. This extraordinary early nineteenth-century American was the daughter of an Episcopal clergyman. After raising her five children, she had converted to Catholicism, founded the American Order of the Sisters of Charity in 1913, and laid the foundations for the American parochial school system.

The first native-born American to be canonized, Mother Seton was declared a saint for two miracles attributed to her. The first reportedly occurred in a young nurse who had widespread cancer; her nurse colleagues had all prayed to Mother Seton for the woman to get well, and she did. We do not know the medical details of that case. The second miracle, however, occurred in a young child who was treated in Baltimore in the early 1950s for acute leukemia and who afterwards was bleeding quite profusely. According to the story, the doctors had indicated that there was nothing more that they could do. The nurses prayed to Mother Seton and the child got well. Before his lecture, Joe talked to the doctor who had made a house call on the child. He learned that the child was suffering from an overdose of the chemotherapy treatment and indeed was bleeding severely owing to the drug side effects that temporarily lowered blood platelet counts. The father was holding the child and crying out, "You're going to die, you're going to die," and the child was yelling right back, "But I don't want to die, I don't want to die!" The doctor sent the child back to St. Agnes Hospital, where she recovered, presumably because the toxicity from the drug wore off, as it usually did. Thereafter the leukemic cells did not recur, and she became a long-term survivor. Different people claimed success for her survival, some pointing to the medical therapy, others to the intercession of Mother Seton, depending on their point of view.

After hearing of these cases, Joe immediately contacted all his friends in the field of hematology who had experience with the chemotherapy of leukemia and quickly found about fifteen other long-term survivors, whose cases he summarized in his lecture. He followed this up with a questionnaire that year to all of the members of the American Society of Hematology and the International Society of Hematology. By correspondence with the doctors who replied, Joe was able to collect follow-up information on 127 surviving patients and to show that indeed, most of them had been cured, as defined by very long (more than five-year) remissions. Most of the patients who were in that category had been treated with 6-MP plus cortisone, 6-MP alone, methotrexate alone or with 6-MP or cortisone, or steroids (cortisone) alone.

This data provided perhaps the first reasonably convincing evidence that acute leukemia was at least occasionally curable, although many in the medical profession remained skeptical. Up until then, the possibility of curing leukemia had not been taken at all seriously.

All of us working in the field have continued to hear statements like, "You'll never cure cancer until you understand the inner workings of the cancer cell," or even, "Cancer is as basic as life itself." Burchenal's consistent response has been: "Yes, you're right, we'll do better in the next century when we know more about these things, but in the meantime we have patients to treat. Cancer has many causes and therefore many treatments will be necessary. In this sense I compare it to infectious disease, which also has many causes and many different types of treatments. Overall I'm reasonably happy with the progress that we have made in cancer chemotherapy, and there are many other success stories in addition to acute leukemia."

One of the traits that was essential to the early chemotherapists was optimism: they had to be optimistic to undertake and persist in such work. But that optimism had to be bolstered by active research programs that allowed them to see that they were learning things, making progress, even if only slowly. Joe recalls: "When the folate antagonists were the only drugs available to produce even a temporary remission, we hoped for something new to come along—and it did in 6-MP." There were a great number of new compounds coming along, and there still are.

Investigators like Burchenal have their own hopefulness raised by the optimism of the patients and their families. When patients and families are presented with a proposal for an experiment with a new drug, they are almost invariably enthusiastic. They welcome the opportunity of participating in something that might benefit them or, at least, yield knowledge that will help others in the future. After all, someone has to be the first to get the drug, and that someone may be the first person on earth to be cured.

When the trial works, the joy for everyone is overwhelming. Joe remembered, for example, one such occasion when Dr. Gerald Rosen and he treated a patient with bone cancer who was the son of a friend. At that time they were just starting to add cisplatin to the complicated adjuvant therapy regimen, which had the disadvantage that it caused a great deal of toxicity. The boy had almost unbearable nausea and vomiting from cisplatin chemotherapy, but his mother begged and cajoled him to remain on the chemotherapy program. Today that young man is cured and has finished college. These are the kinds of exciting leads that pose real opportunities for better treatment.

Another patient, a college student whose leukemic tumor went into remission, sent Joe a photograph of herself sitting on top of a Swiss alp that she had climbed: "You can imagine how that made me feel!"

One of the great stories of the treatment of leukemia also derives in part from Joe's labors. The chemotherapy work that he was doing in children with leukemia led him and his associates to the discovery of a successful treatment for lymphoma in Africa, the so-called Burkitt lymphoma that is common in children living in East Africa. This is a highly malignant disease of lymphocytes, much like childhood acute lymphocytic leukemia, but with a somewhat different clinical presentation. The curability of such patients was clearly a by-product of the leukemia research program. Burchenal has consistently taught that the study of leukemia is particularly productive because this disease is a stalking horse for cancer chemotherapy. The principles useful in leukemia are often applicable and effective in the treatment of other diseases.

CHAPTER 5

George H. Hitchings, Ph.D.

A greater, more lasting and far-reaching glory,
that of service to his fellow man.
—George Hitchings (credo at age 17)

On my way to work on October 17, 1988, I almost crashed the car with excitement when the radio announced that my friends, George Hitchings and Gertrude Elion, had been awarded the Nobel Prize for Medicine and Physiology. It was a fitting cap to their scientific careers; nonetheless, it was a surprise to me and to them: Nobel Prizes are rarely given to cancer researchers, much less to those who work in drug development. The prize recognized both a major intellectual achievement—figuring out how to design new drugs to block specific metabolic pathways in misbehaving cells—and the successful application of that insight against acute leukemia and a host of other terrible diseases.

The older partner of this remarkable team of researchers, George Hitchings, was born in 1905 in Hoquian, Washington, and spent most of his childhood in Bellingham, where his father supervised the building of a fleet of ships for the PacificAmerican Fisheries Company. The elder Hitchings had been the primary architect of the transition from wooden hull sailing ships to steam vessels. A craftsman with wood, he had built all sorts of toys for little George. He served as a source of inspiration to his young son, but for all too brief a time. He died a lingering death from an infection following a delayed appendectomy.

When George was growing up, he was often told that, if he got to be as good a man as his father, he'd be a great success. He learned only late in his life from his older sister that, when he was baptized, his father had held him up and dedicated his life to the service of mankind. His father, revered in his community for his good works, would have been proud to know that his son contributed so directly to the vitality of science and to the health of the nation. George likes to tell people that, at the time he was born, the average life expectancy in the United States was forty-six years. Health research was to increase that dramatically, by an additional thirty years, and—though George is too modest to say so—his share of the research contributed in significant ways to that lengthened life span.

George Hitchings attended an excellent grade school, run by the Bellingham Teachers College and notable for its enthusiastic, young teachers. George remembers taking a poll in class for the presidential candidates, Hughes versus Wilson, and chalking the results up on the blackboard, possibly his first effort at quantifying data. An eighth-grade English teacher at Leschi School in Seattle, Winona Proper, instilled in George a lasting appreciation for Shakespeare and for precision in the use of language. As salutatorian at Franklin High School, he presented a brief biography of Louis Pasteur. In his address, he characterized Pasteur as having achieved "a greater, more lasting and far-reaching glory, that of service to his fellow man"—a credo that has always been his own as well. Pasteur became George's role model because he was not only a great scientist but a humanitarian. "I've always had two aspects in mind—scientific achievement and humanitarianism. That makes a well-rounded life. That's my philosophy, two-thirds science and one-third philanthropy."

George entered the University of Washington as a premedical student, but during his first year he became enchanted with chemistry and ended up majoring in the subject with a minor in humanities. That combination made him a "queer bird" among the chemistry majors because he took so many language, humanities, and social science courses. Later on, his love of humanities was greatly enriched by the love and creative talents of his wife, Beverly, a skilled teacher who wrote, painted, and, by way of relaxation, designed and made all of her own clothing. She didn't make her husband's clothing, however, and George seldom shopped for clothes. From his early days in college onward, he often wore suits and trousers full of nitric acid holes—the proud badge of an old-time chemist.

After completing his B.S. degree, George did research at Puget Sound Biological Station. He spent a wonderful summer on the lab's oceanographic vessel learning from the many scientists who were studying the fish and waters of the Sound. George wrote his first two scientific papers then. "Chemistry of the Waters of Argyle Lagoon" explained why the density and salt content of water in various parts of the lagoon varied so much. Water in the deeper parts of the lagoon did not mix as readily as did the water in the shallower parts. The explanation was really quite simple, George felt; nonetheless the experience of doing original research was very satisfying.

His next stop was Harvard University's graduate school in 1928. He spent a year in Cambridge as a chemistry major and then moved across the Charles River to work in the Department of Biological Chemistry at the Harvard Medical School with Dr. Otto Folin and with Dr. Cyrus Fiske, his Ph.D. advisor. At the time Fiske was in the process of describing adenosine triphosphate (ATP), a major "currency" in the transfer of chemical energy in cell metabolism. George's work with Fiske on this major problem eventually led him to study other nucleic acids.

Unfortunately, Dr. Fiske was near the end of his own career and was not an effective supervisor. Without his advisor's cooperation, George could not publish anything on the experiments he'd done jointly with Fiske— even his thesis work did not appear in print for some six years after he received his Ph.D. in 1933. George graduated during the depths of the Depression, and his lack of scientific publications made him a weak candidate for the very few available jobs. Even the prestige of a Harvard degree could not compensate for this deficiency. The next nine years were very hard. George had to make do with fellowships and odd jobs, culminating in an unhappy year at Western Reserve Medical School in Cleveland. While he was at Western Reserve, a colleague persuaded him to join Burroughs Wellcome, a pharmaceutical company then located in Tuckahoe, New York.

George and Beverly had met at Harvard, gotten married in graduate school, and began their family not long after he joined Burroughs Wellcome in 1942—first a daughter and then a son, Tom. During the course of Tom's gestation, it was discovered that George and Beverly had an Rh blood group incompatibility. Beverly was fortunate to carry Tom to full term, but they were aware from the seventh month on that the baby was going to have jaundice, anemia, and possible brain damage from a dread disease called erythroblastosis foetalis. Tom was one of the very first babies in the world to be treated for this by an exchange transfusion. The inventor of the technique, Dr. Alex Weiner, came up from Long Island with tubes of donated blood. George centrifuged the blood for Dr. Weiner, and they passed the tubes of blood back and forth to each other during the transfusion.

The tasks for the anxious scientist-father continued in the days that followed as George kept track of Tom's blood counts. At last Tom began to make healthy blood on his own. One day George held Tom up to a mirror, and the five-month-old child looked at his reflection and said, "Pretty baby"—astounding his parents and just about everybody else. George and Beverly had been worried about the possibility of brain damage, but when they heard Tom speak, their fears were put to rest. George was the beneficiary of a new medical discovery; soon others would benefit from his discoveries.

When George started work at Burroughs Wellcome, he *was* the Biochemistry Department. The administration let young Dr. Hitchings develop his own program. Chemotherapy, that is, the use of drugs to achieve cures, was then in its infancy. It consisted largely of trial-and-error testing done by the pharmaceutical industry. According to the prevailing practice, compounds would be chosen more or less at random and injected into some type of biological system, such as an infected mouse, with the hope that something useful would be discovered that would lead to the development of a new drug.

Scientists in academia stood disdainfully apart from this kind of activity and argued that it would be premature to attempt chemotherapy without sufficient basic knowledge about biochemistry, physiology, and pharmacology. In truth, the field had been sterile for thirty-five years or so since Ehrlich's work. No new agents of any importance had been developed. But the discovery of sulfonamides and development of the drug Prontosil in 1942 changed the field of pharmacology forever. Not only did the heroes of the sulfa drug story—Gerhard Domagk, D. D. Woods, Paul Fildes— come up with a drug that could halt otherwise fatal infections, but they also came up with a persuasive explanation of why it worked.

Domagk, Woods, and Fildes showed that Prontosil blocked a nutrient that was key to the bacteria's metabolism. If the bacterial cell could not absorb this nutrient, it could not grow and reproduce, and so it could not harm the human host. Such key nutrients—crucial links in the chains of biochemical reactions that make up a cell's metabolism—are called *metabolites*. Thus Prontosil was an antimetabolite.

It turned out that the particular metabolite blocked by the drug was a previously unknown nutrient, folic acid, and that folic acid was essential to the synthesis of the nucleic acids, DNA and RNA, in all living cells. (Folic acid's role in the formation of red blood cells and the prevention of anemia was only discovered later.) The discovery of folic acid and its function around 1945 focused new attention on the role of the mysterious nucleic acids. The nucleic acids were obviously vitally important (every cell contained them), yet no one knew what they did. This was, mind you, long before Watson and Crick's 1953 publication of the double-helix structure of DNA and its function as the carrier of genetic information.

For the time being, it was the whole notion of antimetabolites that captured George Hitchings's imagination. If you could find or create antimetabolites that would block specific metabolic systems—whether these were pathways essential to the infecting organism or pathways that somehow went awry in the human body—then you had some hope of halting or even reversing the disease process. The possibilities were as vast and exciting as biology itself, and George never looked back. "I reasoned that, since sulfa drugs could be antimetabolites against bacteria, perhaps we could make other substances that were similar to normal nucleic acids and yet sufficiently different that they might inhibit the growth of bacteria and possibly also tumors."

The theory of antimetabolites was simple enough. To make one, you synthesize a compound whose chemical structure is so similar to a normal metabolite or nutrient that it fools the cell into thinking it's the real thing. The cell then takes up this antimetabolite as if it were the normal metabolite and incorporates it into the machinery of the cell. But because of that small but critical difference in the chemical structure, sooner or later the antimetabolite becomes the monkey wrench that jams up the works. Or, to change the metaphor, it becomes the counterfeit coin that goes in the vending machine and then gets stuck and stops the whole machine from working.

To put the theory into practice, however, would take incredible amounts of patience, meticulous care, unflagging energy, biological and chemical insight, imagination, organization, luck, and lots of money. George Hitchings, his colleagues, and his company had them all.

Today, biochemistry laboratory walls are likely to sport enormous charts depicting the metabolic pathways of the cell—incredibly complex, interconnecting loops, cycles, and chains of the chemical reactions needed to sustain life. Interfere with any step in any reaction, and the consequences may show up in pathways that seem remote in function from the disrupted one. When Hitchings started work on antimetabolites in the late 1940s, these detailed road maps of cell metabolism did not exist. Some metabolic cycles and cascades had been elucidated in their main outlines, but it was obvious that dozens more remained to be discovered, worked out in detail, and their interactions explored. The map was essentially blank. How then to identify and isolate those pathways that particularly interested you and to pinpoint each step?

The key to any physiological experiment is to set up a model system in which you can control and manipulate the pertinent factors. The choice of experimental organism as biological model is crucial. George decided to use two species of bacteria. Bacteria had several advantages as experimental material; they were small, fast-growing living cells, relatively easy to culture, maintain, measure, and medically important. The two different species served as checks on each other.

George and his first recruit, Elvira Falco, a college graduate interested in science, began by determining the bacteria's bare nutritional requirements for growth, a difficult task in itself. Once they found reliable growth media that would enable them to raise bacteria in strictly controlled conditions, they could move on to the next step: adding the compound they had synthesized in the hope that it would act as an inhibitor, that is, as an antimetabolite. If the compound was indeed a true antimetabolite, then its inhibiting effect on the cell's growth could be bypassed by adding extra quantities of the nutrient it had blocked.

These painstaking experiments had to be done methodically, in duplicate or triplicate, over weeks and months. Hitchings and Falco had to ensure that each new result was not accidental before going on to the next step. The lab was full of round Petri dishes, each with its blobs of bacterial colonies—and each bearing notations of what growth factors were in the original culture medium and what inhibitor had been added. Planning the experiments and interpreting the results was like doing a diagramless crossword puzzle, where you could not even be sure what the letters of the alphabet were.

The test system was biological, the inhibitors were created with the tools of organic chemistry, and the experimental design and analyses were a matter of logic. This blending of disciplines was novel and refreshing: George liked to call it "enlightened empiricism." Creating this *method* for the study of metabolites and their antagonists was as important as the growth factors and inhibitory drugs it revealed. Indeed, the method remains in use by many scientists, long after some of the drugs have been replaced by better ones.

In 1944 the department grew to include Gertrude (Trudy) Elion, who is the subject of Chapter 6. Her first project was to try to create drugs that would inhibit overactive thyroid glands, that is, to find a treatment for hyperthyroidism. At that she was not successful. Each new chemical compound Trudy synthesized became grist for trials with the bacterial growth assay system. Even if a compound was completely ineffective at quelling hyperthyroidism, it might be a useful antimetabolite for some other illness.

George's initial fascination was with discovering nutrients that facilitated the synthesis of nucleic acids and with antimetabolites that interfered with or jammed their synthesis. The little group focused on one small yet complex part of nucleic acid synthesis: the purines. Two purine compounds, guanine and adenine, were known to be essential building blocks in the synthesis of DNA (although precisely how these compounds fit together would not be clear until Watson and Crick's work a few years later). If you tinkered with the basic structure of those two purines, adding side chains or otherwise slightly modifying them chemically, the new purine-related compounds ought to act as antimetabolites to bacterial DNA synthesis and hence to stop cell growth. By the mid-1940s Hitchings and Falco showed that a variety of purine antimetabolites could hinder the growth of such killer bacteria as *Staphylococcus* and coliform organisms. They also appreciated the more general point: antimetabolites were really directed against *any* rapidly growing cell, any cell where new DNA was being synthesized quickly. So cells that grew more rapidly than normal—that is, cancer cells—ought to be especially vulnerable to these new chemicals.

In 1947 the Burroughs Wellcome team began trying out their experimental compounds against experimentally induced cancers in mice. C. P. Rhoads at Memorial Sloan-Kettering in New York City had been collecting all sorts of drugs and chemical agents from many sources to test on mouse tumors. George sent four compounds, including a purine antimetabolite synthesized by Trudy Elion. This compound, 2,6-diaminopurine, attracted Rhoads's attention when it inhibited first one kind of mouse tumor, then several others as well. Joe Burchenal quickly tried it out clinically. By 1948, George Hitchings was hooked on cancer research as a career. The clincher came when the biochemist learned that a twenty-three-year-old woman suffering from acute lymphoblastic leukemia had experienced a complete remission after treatment with 2,6-diaminopurine.

"What a feeling of elation this was! Many months later I heard from Joe Burchenal that she was still in remission and she had had a baby. But everyone else was telling Joe this patient must not have had acute leukemia or else she surely would have died, that being the conventional wisdom of the time. Sadly, she confirmed the correctness of the diagnosis: she relapsed with her leukemia and ultimately did die. Unfortunately too, there was no way of continuing to treat her, because we had no other drugs and we couldn't continue to use 2,6-diaminopurine because it was too toxic. That was the limitation of our knowledge at that time." But they had had a glimpse of the promised land.

Basic scientists such as George Hitchings rarely have an opportunity to follow their discoveries into the clinic and to learn what happens to individual patients who might benefit from their stubborn, step-by-step advances in laboratory research. In this case, the communication between the basic scientist George Hitchings and the clinician Joseph Burchenal was very close, and the basic scientist had a taste of the excitement a clinical researcher feels when an experiment with real patients turns out successfully.

Hitchings, Falco, and Elion renewed the search for variations on the purine theme, trying to synthesize other compounds that would share or improve on 2,6-diaminopurine's effectiveness but reduce its toxicity. In 1951 Trudy Elion, adapting a tricky chemical reaction that Elvira Falco had worked out earlier, succeeded in synthesizing a new purine that looked just like a normal metabolite, hypoxanthine, except that it had a sulphur group stuck onto one corner of the purine ring. The new antimetabolite, 6-mercaptopurine—or, as it was quickly abbreviated, 6-MP—turned out to be a vital key to chemotherapy for leukemia for decades to come.

When Hitchings tested 6-MP in the bacterial growth assay system, the compound did precisely what they hoped. The bacteria's growth was indeed strongly inhibited by 6-MP; adding back the blocked normal metabolite, hypoxanthine, restored normal growth. Hitchings gave the Memorial Sloan-Kettering researchers 6-MP along with a whole series of related compounds to try out on the experimental mice tumors. From that batch of compounds, the eight that brought about immediate shrinkage of mouse cancers were selected for testing on patients. That first cut left out 6-MP. But then the researchers looked again at the mice that had been treated with 6-MP. Two weeks of treatment with 6-MP—rather than just a week—showed spectacular results: 40 percent of the mouse tumors had disappeared entirely. This had never been seen before in the lab.

Within a year of the synthesis of 6-MP, it had been shown to be active against tumors and leukemia in mice. Within a mere year and a half after its synthesis, Joe Burchenal had taken 6-MP into the clinic and was obtaining remissions with his leukemia patients.

Dr. Rhoads got so excited that he organized a cooperative study of the drug—the first of its kind for cancer chemotherapy. Rhoads sent 6-MP samples to a dozen investigators at other hospitals, and almost all got similar positive results. The one exception, curiously, was Dr. Sidney Farber at Harvard, who never got a remission using 6-MP—an odd counterpoint to the Sloan-Kettering group's difficulty in getting remissions with Farber's first compound, aminopterin.

At that point, 6-MP looked so encouraging that Rhoads persuaded Charles Kettering, the hospital's millionaire patron, to give money directly to Burroughs Wellcome, specially earmarked for the Hitchings program. The discovery of 6-MP and Kettering's donation came just in the nick of time. Hitchings's boss had been on the verge of scaling down the Biochemistry Department and had already issued termination notices to some of the staff in the lab. "We were rescued in the eleventh hour," Hitchings remembers. Such philanthropic support for research in a pharmaceutical firm was (and, as far as Hitchings knows, still is) unique.

In his excitement, Rhoads also talked to reporters, and the story broke in the *New York Daily Mirror*. The famous newscaster Walter Winchell, who was a big supporter of the Damon Runyon Memorial Fund that aided Memorial Sloan-Kettering, was annoyed not to be given the scoop. Nonetheless, on his influential Sunday night radio show, Winchell announced in his dramatic and telegraphic style that Sloan-Kettering scientists had discovered a new treatment for leukemia, a wonder drug synthesized by one Dr. George Hitchings.

In the next few days George was inundated with over six hundred calls from desperate doctors and patients. The Medical Department at Burroughs Wellcome was taken by surprise by this new development; ordinarily they would have been prepared to provide follow-up information about how and where to obtain their drugs. They began to realize that it wasn't fair to create a demand for a life-saving product and not be able to meet the demand. Supplies of 6-MP were extremely limited. The company went full steam ahead to increase the synthesis of the drug, even though it had no idea of what the manufacturing costs would be, how it would distribute the drugs, or how it should respond to the many pathetic appeals it was receiving from dying patients.

The Medical Department quickly filed a New Drug Application with the Food and Drug Administration. George Hitchings now had an experience unique in history: the head of the New Drug Division of the FDA, Dr. King, took it upon himself to evaluate the 6-MP data personally. He visited all the investigators working with this compound and, with astonishing speed, decided that the drug was effective and approved a license in September of 1953. King took this action fully eight months before the clinical results had even been summarized or reported. The drug 6-MP indeed had useful clinical properties. It doubled the otherwise meager life expectancy of children with acute leukemia, and it was even effective in some patients who were resistant to other available agents.

The U.S. Patent Office reacted to 6-MP with equally amazing speed. In order to grant a patent for an anticancer drug, the office normally required data on the so-called five-year cures. This meant that the sponsoring company had to point to patients who had survived for five years and appeared to be cured of their disease. Such a criterion was clearly not feasible for an antileukemia drug, and no one wanted to wait for five years to release 6-MP, given such clear results from the initial treatment. Burroughs Wellcome petitioned the patent examiner, who appealed to his own superior for a waiver. The two officials investigated the situation, set aside their usual rule, and awarded the company the patent.

However, the FDA and Patent Office approvals could not solve Burroughs Wellcome's manufacturing problems. There is a big difference between synthesizing small quantities of a compound in a research laboratory for testing proposals and manufacturing huge batches of pills or ampules to sell commercially to thousands of patients. In the year in which 6-MP was approved, George and his colleagues spent the Christmas holidays making enough of the drug to give to patients. They even spent New Year's Day in the laboratory doing the repetitive, boring drudge work. George recalls that he went off in the morning with a sandwich in his pocket and, at the end of the day, Beverly asked if he was aware that it was New Year's Day. They were trying to do in a small chemical laboratory what would later be done in a factory.

"This entire period was a real emotional roller coaster ride," George recalls. "We would see a half-dead child recover quickly, get out of bed, and go back to school and play baseball, but almost inevitably the child would relapse and die. In fact, we thought that all of the children relapsed. But they didn't. Every once in a while one was cured. This was not discovered until much later and we were not even thinking of the word 'cure.' Once, years later, on a cruise, Beverly and I were having dinner with some people from Houston whose daughter, while a seven-year-old child, had been treated with 6-MP and cortisone and had been cured of her leukemia. By that time she had reached the age of twenty-seven and had three sons. I want to tell you that this is the most rewarding thing that can happen to anybody, more rewarding than papers or prizes. Physicians get a chance to see individual patients survive, but chemists rarely do."

No other cancer chemotherapy drug has ever moved so quickly from the biochemists' lab to the clinic and the hospital pharmacy. The problem is not, George Hitchings observes with considerable bitterness, with the researchers, but with the United States government's procedures for approving drugs. "What happened with 6-MP could never happen today, because every drug we've ever invented, with the exception of 6-MP, has been invented in the United States, yet marketed worldwide for as long as five years before being approved in this country. I'm pretty discouraged about the FDA. It often seems to me that the first thing the government does is give people an IQ test, and anyone who scores over 80 is automatically disqualified for government service."

The dramatic success with 6-MP triggered a whole series of discoveries that exemplify George Hitchings's philosophy of "enlightened empiricism." They also exemplify what George feels is his greatest asset as a scientist: the ability to interpret research data that is available to everyone, find a new meaning for it, and react on that insight. Take, for example, the drug Imuran.

By the time of the 1954 symposium on 6-MP, Trudy Elion had shown that 6-MP was partly inactivated by an enzyme called xanthine oxidase. That is, the enzyme broke down 6-MP so that it was excreted rather than allowed to interfere with the growth of the cancer cells. Perhaps a slight change in the structure of 6-MP would resist the enzyme's attack and thus be more effective than 6-MP. The Burroughs Wellcome team churned out variant after variant of 6-MP, hoping to thwart the enzyme. One of these was originally tagged BW57-322—the three hundred and twenty-second compound made that year, 1957, at Burroughs Wellcome (the tag number alone suggests the pace Hitchings and his colleagues were setting)—and later named Imuran. It seemed that its chemical structure made it less prone to being deactivated by the enzyme and thus its anticancer effects might last longer in patients. I myself participated in some clinical studies (with Dr. R. Wayne Rundles at Duke) on Imuran and showed that the new compound was about as effective as 6-MP, but no better. So the drug was shelved. But then it got a second life.

Dr. Robert Schwartz—a young medical scientist who had taken part of his training with my father in New York—and his senior colleague, Dr. William Dameshek, of Tufts University in Boston, were interested in bone marrow transplantation in humans. But everything that they had tried to prevent the rejection of a transplant had failed. Bob Schwartz reviewed the literature and realized that there was a group of chemotherapeutic drugs that had never been tried and were perhaps worth trying. He knew that antimetabolites had inhibitory effects against young lymphocytes, the types of cells involved in antibody formation. Schwartz therefore wrote to Hitchings and asked for 25 grams of 6-MP and, at the very same time, wrote to Lederle Laboratories and asked them for methotrexate so he could try these two antimetabolite drugs in his bone marrow transplant experiments. George sent his 6-MP by return mail, but somehow Schwartz's letter to Lederle never got to the right place. We now know that, if the events had been reversed—if Bob had been sent the methotrexate from Lederle and not the 6-MP from George—his experiment would have failed, because methotrexate is inactive in that test system. After about a year of research with rabbits, however, Dr. Schwartz was able to show that 6-MP could inhibit the rabbits' antibody response after they had been challenged by a foreign antigen. Schwartz and his colleagues had found a way to prevent antibodies from being formed, a way of stopping an "allergic response." Their article on this exciting discovery came to the attention of Dr. Roy Calne of Great Britain, who was then studying the rejection of transplanted kidneys in dogs. He too obtained some 6-MP and found that dogs that were treated with this drug survived longer than the untreated controls. One survived for forty-six days with a transplanted kidney, as opposed to the ten to twelve days typical without the use of the drug. Young Dr. Calne headed to Peter Bent Brigham Hospital in Boston, then the mecca of kidney transplantation, for additional training. It was the Boston group that had developed the surgical techniques for successfully transplanting kidneys between identical twins. But all attempts, in animals and in humans, to cross the immune barrier with a transplant among non-twins brought about disaster: the transplanted kidney was invariably rejected by the recipient. Investigators at the Brigham Hospital had tried everything they knew to prevent tissue rejection, but nothing worked.

On his way to Boston, Calne visited the Hitchings group to discuss a new approach. When he left Tuckahoe, he carried several compounds in his pockets, including BW57-322. Within a few months he wrote to George that BW57-322 "was not uninteresting." Deciphering this bit of British understatement, George made haste to visit Harvard where he saw the remarkable survival rate among dogs that had been given kidney transplants. One dog, whom Calne had whimsically called Lollipop, carried a foreign kidney from an unrelated dog for many months. The kidney worked so well that she even managed to conceive and bear puppies. Many other dogs had also been treated with BW57-322 and were doing well with their kidney transplants. George asserts today: "I would go so far as to say that without Lollipop we wouldn't have organ transplantation, and terminally ill kidney failure patients are no longer lost after kidney transplants thanks to the technology that includes this important drug."

The drug that Rundles and I had dismissed as no better than 6-MP for leukemia thus proved to be remarkably effective in preventing organ rejection. It is the drug of choice for kidney transplantation and the transplantation of other organs as well. But that's not the only thing this compound turned out to be good for. At about the same time as Calne's success, the group I was in at Duke was finding out that BW57-322 also helped to alleviate a variety of auto-immmune conditions, disorders where, in effect, the body becomes allergic to itself. I remember treating a twenty-three-year-old woman who suffered both from chronic leukemia and a severe auto-immune condition called erythema nodosum. Very painful swollen nodules on her legs and ankles were so tender that she could barely walk. We were trying out Imuran for her leukemia, and the leukemia got better. But so did her erythema nodosum, an improvement that was entirely unexpected. This type of clinical result opened up a whole new approach to the treatment of allergic or auto-immune conditions such as lupus erythematosus, and it was the outgrowth of enlightened empiricism in cancer research.

There was still another card to be played in following up the enzymatic destruction of 6-MP. Suppose, Hitchings and his colleagues argued, we try to inhibit the enzyme that destroys 6-MP. They then "invented" allopurinol, another antimetabolite structure. Allopurinol was intended to make 6-MP more effective against leukemia. Giving allopurinol together with 6-MP meant that smaller doses of 6-MP would achieve the same effect that larger doses would in the absence of allopurinol. It gave 6-MP a more powerful punch but not a better antileukemic effect: that was disappointing. However, it did something else that was remarkable: it inhibited the formation of uric acid in humans. Uric acid is a normal breakdown product of cells; it has to be fully excreted in the urine. If it builds up in the bloodstream, it will cause gout.

How well I remember those studies! The early clinical work was being done by my mentor, Dr. Wayne Rundles, myself, Doctors Earl Metz and Harold Silberman, and junior colleagues at Duke. The metabolic work was being done by Hitchings and Elion, who were still in Tuckahoe, New York, at that time. We used to treat patients who had chronic leukemia, making very careful clinical measurements of all of their blood counts, chemistries, and the size of the liver and spleen, which were generally quite enlarged. We also collected 24-hour urine samples on each patient every day and measured out a portion to send periodically to the Burroughs Wellcome laboratories for analysis. We had a black leather satchel into which the ice-chilled urine samples were put, and I occasionally transported a precious satchel by airplane from Durham to LaGuardia Airport to make sure that these particularly valuable samples didn't get broken. A driver would be sent to meet the plane and take the refrigerated samples on to Tuckahoe.

I had to learn the art of collecting 24-hour urine samples from patients who were in the hospital, something that is much harder than you would think. Either the patient would forget to collect a urine sample, the nurses would discard it, or some other accident would happen to make the collection incomplete. Dr. Rundles and I were treating a delightful elderly woman who had chronic leukemia and who had agreed to take one of George's experimental drugs. Dr. Rundles explained the procedure to her very carefully, and he particularly emphasized the quantitative urine collection. He repeatedly explained to her that at 7:00 A.M. on the next morning she would urinate and discard the sample into the commode; from that time on she would collect every drop of urine into the bottle up until 7:00 A.M the following morning, when she would again void and add that as the final sample to the 24-hour collection. He rehearsed this with her and explained that if she left the ward for any reason that she had to take the jug with her. She repeated back all of the instructions very accurately. The next morning on rounds, we got there shortly after 7:00 A.M. and she pointed proudly to the urine jug that was in a small refrigerator in her room. Rundles quizzed her about all the samples and made sure that none had been missed. Thus reassured, he gave her another jug and told her that the next 24-hour urine sample collection was beginning immediately and would go just as before, until the next morning at 7:00 A.M. We preceeded back down to the laboratory and were talking about the studies to be done. When we got back, however, he amazed me by pouring the entire 24-hour urine collection down the laboratory sink. I tried to stop him, thinking he was making a mistake, but he said, "No, that one was just for practice, and today the urine collection is for real." I was deeply impressed by this meticulous attention to detail.

While keeping track of all these measurements, we noted that allopurinol profoundly lowered the uric acid level in the blood of our patients. One day, while reviewing the chart of a patient, we joked that, although allopurinol didn't seem to be very useful in leukemia, maybe it would be useful in treating gout. Our initial patient, who happened to have both gout and leukemia, told us that his arthritis was getting better. People who had severe gouty arthritis, with huge deposits of bony-like uric acid grotesquely deforming the joints of their hands, feet, knees, or elbows, found that these deposits slowly melted away as they took the drug, and their joints improved as they had not for many years. With subsequent studies, allopurinol has proved to be the drug of choice for gout, and it is now widely used around the world.

Most doctors think that the discovery of allopurinol's effectiveness for gout was total serendipity. But it was really the serendipity of the prepared mind—which is, as Pasteur observed, what research is all about. In fact, before the clinical studies of allopurinol were ever initiated, Hitchings had very much in mind the knowledge that the enzyme xanthine oxidase's function in the body was not the breakdown of an artificial antimetabolite like 6-MP but, rather, to assist in the metabolic reactions that produced uric acid, the gout-producing waste product. When allopurinol proved to be effective in the Burroughs Wellcome lab at inhibiting xanthine oxidase, he urged Dr. Rundles to measure uric acid in patients treated with the drug. Thus it was no accident that the effect was found—what was lucky was that the effect could be profound and persistent, and could forever change the story of gouty deposits in the joints of afflicted patients.

The Hitchings group had one success after another from 1947 on. In addition to the drugs already mentioned, they discovered trimethoprin (Daraprim) for malaria and the potent antibiotic Septra. Acyclovir (Zovirax), discovered by Trudy Elion, was the first major drug to be effective against viruses, notably the herpes virus. AIDS drugs came later.

Looking back on his career at Burroughs Wellcome, George Hitchings has mixed feelings: profound gratitude for the latitude he had to pursue his research, but annoyance at the company's reluctance to reward him for his immense contributions. More than most pharmaceutical companies, Burroughs Wellcome could afford to let George work out his scientific discoveries even if he could not point to immediate marketable results. George likes to quote the rule of the company's founder, Sir Henry Wellcome: "If you have an idea, I'll give you the freedom to develop it." Because Wellcome set up the company largely as a nonprofit enterprise, and its "profits" go into a foundation for medical research, the pressure for quick payoffs from research is not as strong as at a conventional pharmaceutical company. A good thing, for the first productive drug George came up with—the antimalarial compound Daraprim—took nine years to develop before it went on the market in 1951.

Nonetheless, George feels no great love for "administrators and their thick-headedness." Although the drugs George has been directly responsible for developing have generated more than $5 million in earnings for the company, George had to fight more than once for the continued existence of his department, its staff, and its programs. "In fact I never had more than part of a normal salary throughout my entire career, which I felt was punishment for being so independent. At one point in my career as a department chairman, I was earning $40,000 a year, while another department chairman at the company was earning $100,000 a year. It was at this time that Beverly and I were spending over a third of our income for the education of our children, but I was too proud to ask for more money. We lived rather frugally and I suppose I first realized this when my daughter was surprised to find me wearing a new suit. The company did move from Tuckahoe to the Research Triangle Park in North Carolina, and I eventually rose to become vice president. At that time my salary was $75,000, but it was without any retirement benefits because by then I was over the age of 65. Fortunately I achieved some financial success after I retired and learned to invest my savings."

It's entirely typical of George Hitchings that his retirement years have been as active, as intellectually fruitful, and as good for humanity as his earlier career. As a hobby, he has become an officer in five different foundations and has created one of his own, to honor his late wife, Beverly. The Greater Triangle Community Service Foundation began in 1983 with George's seed money of $1,000 and has grown to hold assets of over $6.5 million. Sadly, Beverly did not live to share George's joy in winning the Nobel Prize, but she would have cheered his decision to use his share of the award to coordinate other local charities' efforts to help community development. George celebrated his second marriage, to Joyce Shaver, M.D.—who works with teenage drug addicts—by setting up a fund to support education about substance abuse.

At the same time, George continues to go to the lab every day to pursue a line of research that has fascinated him ever since he worked on antimalarial drugs in the 1940s. Why are these compounds so highly selective: devastating one strain of bacteria or parasite, leaving another unscathed? It took George years to convince administrators that different species of organisms have enough differences in their metabolisms that it is possible to target and inhibit an enzyme of a particular micro-organism without causing major damage to its animal or human host. "Understanding the biochemical basis of species' differences is turning out to be more remarkable than ever, now that we understand the molecular basis of the differences between enzymes from various species. I'm busily working on new x-ray crystallographic techniques which make it possible to visualize the interaction between drugs and their enzyme target. This is very exciting work which will make it easier to design compounds to do specific tasks and inhibit specific reactions within the cell."

It is absolutely fitting that George's Nobel Prize in 1988 was capped by an even rarer honor the next year: the Albert Schweitzer Prize. It is awarded only once every four years, after a worldwide search, to individuals who show excellence in science or humanities and share Dr. Schweitzer's "reverence for life" in their commitment to humanitariasim. George set out on that path of "service to his fellow man" as a high school salutatorian. Few can claim to have done it so well for so long.

CHAPTER 6

Gertrude B. Elion, Ph.D. (Hon.)

Chance favors only the mind that is prepared.
—*Louis Pasteur*

Until recently, women who have been recognized for making major contributions to the basic sciences have been uncommon. In chemistry they have been decidedly rare. Nor was there anything obvious in the early beginnings of Gertrude Elion's scientific career to provide a clue that she might someday share the Nobel Prize with her lifelong colleague George Hitchings. As a chemist, pharmacologist, and student of biology, Trudy has contributed greatly to the treatment of leukemia and numerous other diseases, and she has been a role model for women scientists in a characteristically male-dominated profession. Chemistry's status as a male preserve made it not a particularly easy profession for her to follow—she had to be powerfully motivated as well as talented. I don't claim to be unbiased, since we have been friends for many years, but everyone who knows her would certainly share those views.

It is difficult to sort out the important factors that go into making career decisions. For Trudy there were two family influences that are worthy of note. One was her grandfather's death from cancer when she was fifteen. "It became my dream to find a cure for cancer. That's the kind of a romantic notion a teenager would have, but it never left me." The second significant factor occured when Trudy was between jobs, early in her professional life. Her father asked if she had ever thought of applying to the Burroughs Wellcome Company, which was in Tuckahoe, near their home. She hadn't ever heard of Burroughs Wellcome, but the suggestion proved to be a turning point in her life. There was to be more good luck in gaining the job.

Trudy earned her bachelor's degree summa cum laude from Hunter College and a master's degree in organic chemistry at New York University. Armed with these two degrees she set out to find work during the second wave of the Depression, in 1937. We have seen how limited employment opportunities were at this time for George, who was experiencing similar difficulties independently. But this was a particularly difficult time for women chemists, and Trudy repeatedly heard that companies to which she was applying had never before hired a chemist of her gender. She began working for the Denver Chemical Manufacturing Company as a chemist's lab assistant in a position where she received no income. She then taught at New York High School as a substitute teacher in chemistry and physics. She finally went to work for Quaker Maid, doing quality control analyses of their food products slated to go to the A & P Food Stores. Later she was hired by Johnson & Johnson in New Brunswick, New Jersey, in a job in which she was synthesizing different sulfonamide derivatives to find one that was more effective. During this time, she was living in the Bronx and commuting about two hours each way. When that project terminated she was again out in the job market.

Trudy then learned about Burroughs Wellcome from her father, who was a dentist and had often received samples from the company. She made an appointment for an interview on a Saturday morning. Burroughs Wellcome (BW) had half of its staff working on Saturdays, it being wartime. It so happened that Dr. Hitchings was at work on that particular Saturday.

"I shudder to think that had I come on an alternate Saturday I might never have gone to Burroughs Wellcome," Trudy recalls. George was not deterred by her lack of a Ph.D., believing her scholastic record showed she could do the work. Nor was he put off by the fact that she was a woman; she was to become the second woman in a laboratory of only three people. "We all worked as equals and we worked very hard." Trudy remembers that even in that first interview George talked with her about his interest in the building blocks of nucleic acid synthesis, the purines, and pyrimidines, and she found this quite exciting though she knew little about the topic. It was this excitment about the science and the opportunity to learn about this area of chemistry that stimulated her to accept the Burroughs Wellcome job in preference to two other job offers which, as luck would have it, happened to come in on the very same day. "That was quite a day."

During her first four years of work at BW, she took graduate courses at night, working toward a Ph.D. degree at Brooklyn Polytechnic Institute. When the dean told her that she would have to give up her job and continue school on a full-time basis in order to get her degree, Trudy had to make a difficult decision. She chose to forget about the Ph.D. and devote all of her energies to work. Of course this turned out to be a most fortunate decision for her (and tough luck on Brooklyn Polytech), but it was a hard choice to make at the time. Trudy has always been sad that neither of her parents lived to see her earn her first honorary doctorate degree and receive the distinguished Garban Medal from the American Chemical Society in 1968, and of course later on the Nobel Prize. Both of her parents had been very supportive of her education and perfectly willing to let her pursue a career that wasn't "acceptable" for women in those days. "I know how much they regretted being unable to finance my graduate education to its completion, and I would so much have wanted to show them that I had succeeded in proving myself to my peers, even without a Ph.D. degree." She was proud to be able to make a gift of $500,000 to Hunter College for a scholarship fund.

Her first assignment at BW, as mentioned earlier, was to begin work on drugs designed to inhibit the function of overactive thyroid glands. This involved synthesizing derivatives of pyrimidines and purines. The idea was to make structural analogs that would look like the real thing to the cell, which would then incorporate the analog and thereby destroy itself. There are classes of drugs that do work precisely in this way to inhibit the thyroid. Her first big excitement, however, came when she synthesized 2,6-diaminopurine. This was found to have strong antibacterial activity in the system that George had worked out. As we heard earlier, this compound was given to Dr. Burchenal, and he and his colleagues found that it inhibited cancers in mice. He quickly tried it in patients, including four who had leukemia. It did have some inhibitory effects against the disease, but it also caused such severe nausea and vomiting that it was clearly not a practical agent. Elion and Hitchings worked hard to develop a way to give the drug intravenously instead of orally, thinking that it might cause less irritation to the bowel, but it still caused similar toxicity.

Knowing that the number six position on the purine chemical ring was a sensitive place in terms of making analogs, Trudy tried to add a chlorine group, but found this extremely difficult to do. Then she read about a new procedure by which an oxygen atom might be replaced by a sulfur atom in that position. She developed a method, and it worked. Her first derivative was thioguanine, *thio* standing for sulfur and *guanine* for the normal purine—hence she developed a normal purine with the substitute of a sulfur group on it to make it into an analog. Once the sulfur was substituted for oxygen on the number six position of that carbon ring, a normal metabolite would convert into an antimetabolite—a critical finding in itself. Thioguanine was still very difficult to purify at this time.

The next compound of this type that she synthesized was 6-mercapto-purine (6-MP), and this of course was the drug that introduced that whole class of chemical derivatives as important antimetabolites. Trudy and George stayed in close contact with Dr. Burchenal with regard to the patients being treated with their compound, but they weren't really able to see patients very often. They felt that they were right on the edge of making a breakthrough, and the experience was an "emotional roller coaster" for doctors, patients, and researchers alike. "We would learn about patients who would have a remission, and then ultimately they would relapse and die. At that time, we thought that we were very close to having the answer for the treatment of leukemia, but that of course turned out to be much further down the road."

It is noteworthy that Trudy describes her contact with patients as an emotional roller coaster, because very similar observations have been made by George and most of the other scientists who participated in the quest for a cure for leukemia. But Trudy and George, with their enlightened empiricism, learned from each of their experiments—no matter whether they turned out positively or negatively.

I remember so well doing collaborative experiments with one of the compounds that Trudy had synthesized, 6-propylmercaptopurine, which I was studying in the laboratory at Duke against human leukemic cells growing in a flask. This chemical was another kind of derivative of the purine ring. It involved adding a three-carbon group plus a sulfur at the six position instead of just a sulfur group, and it has been found to be very active against mouse cancers. Trudy's team had found it to be an extremely potent inhibitor of cancers in mice. I found it to be a tremendous inhibitor of the metabolism of human leukemic cells, and we were very excited at the thought that this might be a powerful antitumor agent in patients.

Then we treated several patients with this drug and absolutely nothing happened to their leukemia. But the first two patients that we treated kept complaining of a garlic odor on their breath, and Dr. Rundles and I had no trouble verifying that observation. When Trudy analyzed the 24-hour urine samples that we collected from these patients, she discovered a unique pathway that occured in humans that did not exist in mice. She learned that our patients were splitting off the three-carbon (propyl) and sulfur group away from the six-carbon purine ring, leaving a normal metabolite plus something called propylmercaptan, which is the essence of garlic. It turned out that mice didn't do that because mouse liver lacks the enzymes that split that compound in precisely that way; thus mice bearing tumors were nicely inhibited by this metabolic inhibitor, as were isolated human leukemic cells. Humans, however, detoxified the compound in the liver into an inert purine and to "garlic," which certainly didn't hurt cancer cells. On that occasion Trudy discovered a pathway that hadn't been known before, and she discovered why a drug didn't work. But many other times she found out why drugs *did* work. That was one of the great strengths of the Elion and Hitchings operation. It was never a hit-or-miss proposition. There was always a question, there was always a hypothesis, and there was usually an answer. And sometimes an answer they had not expected.

Trudy is modest in talking about her accomplishments; she would rather talk about an opera, or a trip, or her family. When pressed about her successes she talks about the importance of serendipity. In doing so, it is interesting that she goes back to the same story about kidney transplantation that George Hitchings referred to. She talks about yet another aspect of that story being a critical factor determined by chance. When Dr. Roy Calne and a colleague from the United Kingdom did get the 6-MP from them, as we heard from George earlier, they divided up the work. His colleague would try to see if the drug prolonged the survival of transplanted skin in mice, and Calne would use it in kidney transplants in dogs. As luck would have it, the colleague went off on a holiday. Instead of waiting for the skin work to be done first, which would have been the natural order of experiments, Calne went ahead and did the kidney transplants and found that 6-MP prolonged the survival of the kidney grafts in the treated animals. When his colleague came back, he independently did the experiments on mice and found no prolongation in the survival of skin grafts transplanted from one mouse strain to another, despite their treatment with 6-MP. Consequently he called Calne and said, "Don't waste your time, because this approach won't work"—but of course, it already had worked. It is a curious fact that 6-MP, its follow-up drug Imuran, and other related drugs do not prolong the grafting of skin, whereas they do prolong the grafting of kidneys. Even today, the explanation for the differences between these effects is not known.

Speaking of luck, most scientists would consider themselves extremely lucky to have made a contribution to the treatment of leukemia or to organ transplantation. But Trudy and George participated in a major way in the treatment of gout, malaria, and bacterial infections, as well. Trudy also developed Zovirax, the first effective treatment of herpes virus infection. "One of the exciting things about my work at BW was that we always seemed to be breaking new ground and trying to learn from our experimental results to unravel some of Nature's secrets. The ability to combine chemistry and biological reactions, and to study the pharmacology of drugs and their effects on the metabolism of tumor cells and bacterial cells, made the work even more interesting and stimulating. There was always so much to learn, so many possible fields in which our findings might be applied. We were learning about new enzymes involved in the synthesis of nucleic acids, and it was particularly satisfying to see how well some of our hypotheses fit into the new knowledge. The feeling of achievement which comes from playing a part in the development of new drugs is so rewarding that I can think of nothing which could be comparable. Every leukemia remission in a child, every successful kidney transplant, every resolution of gouty joints destroyed by uric acid, every relief from suffering in people with herpes infections—all are deep, personal satisfactions. I feel so fortunate to have had the opportunity to have fulfilled so many hopes and dreams, even if not all of them."

PART III

The Hub

NCI

In its heyday, the hub of cancer research in the world was unquestionably the National Cancer Institute (NCI) and its Clinical Center in Bethesda, Maryland. At its modern beginnings in 1953, though, NCI and its parent, the National Institutes of Health (NIH), started with nothing but a collection of brand-new laboratories and its Clinical Center, a young, inexperienced staff, and an extraordinary vision of the future of biomedical research. The primary goal of NIH's founders—a determined group of physicians, scientists, influential lay people, and members of Congress—was to found an institution that would use research to create knowledge toward the cure of major diseases. They believed that the best way to encourage first-rate research would be to bring together a critical mass of bright, dedicated young men and women, give them all the resources they needed, and free them from the extraneous tasks of teaching, administration, and routine patient care.

The salaries at NCI were poor compared with those in private practice or industry, but access to lab space, to equipment, to stimulating colleagues, and to patients was unparalleled. NCI made an unheard-of offer of free treatment to patients whose cases fitted into particular research programs. The patients—often desperately ill—came to NCI knowing that the treatment they got would be experimental, that they might not survive any longer than they would with conventional care, but that, by participating in the research, they might help future patients if not themselves. That courageous spirit gave impetus to the doctor-scientists who cared for them and learned from them.

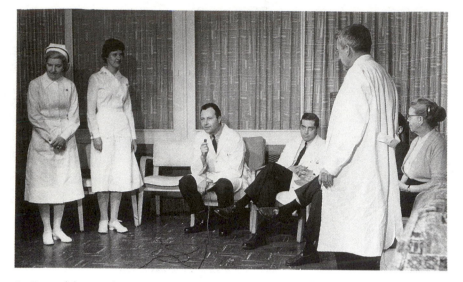

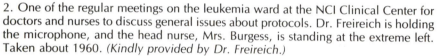

2. One of the regular meetings on the leukemia ward at the NCI Clinical Center for doctors and nurses to discuss general issues about protocols. Dr. Freireich is holding the microphone, and the head nurse, Mrs. Burgess, is standing at the extreme left. Taken about 1960. *(Kindly provided by Dr. Freireich.)*

The NCI began with a small staff of "senior" scientists, all of them new to the study of cancer and leukemia, and most of them not so senior either— some had just a year or two of internship and residency under their belts. They were assisted by a steady stream of even younger physicians who, hoping for careers in medical research, did their military service as two-year NCI clinical associates with a formal rank of senior assistant surgeons in the U.S. Public Health Service. Under the leadership of Dr. C. Gordon Zubrod, the clinical director of the NCI, these novice scientists shaped the discipline of cancer research during the 1950s and 1960s. Many ultimately became leaders in oncology, the study and treatment of cancer. But in those early days, before oncology was formally recognized as a specialty within medicine and before anyone had any real basis for hoping to cure cancer, it took special dedication for these young doctors to devote their energy, ideas, and careers to the care of people with cancer.

Zubrod's two protégés with the confusingly similar names—Dr. Emil Frei III (known as Tom) and Dr. Emil J Freireich (known as J)—thrived on the unique opportunity to combine experimental research with clinical work. The two young men complemented each other remarkably well: both were extroverted, boisterous, brilliant, and intellectually probing, but Frei was a peacemaker, Freireich a maverick. Together they achieved far more than either one could have on his own. Out of their intense study of the course of their patients' illnesses, their passionate concern for the patients' well-being, and the unremitting interplay of their lively minds and tongues came idea after idea for treating leukemia.

By contrast, their boss, Dr. Zubrod, was a modest, even retiring gentleman, far more sophisticated and scholarly than either of his two brash and ambitious young colleagues. His quiet charm, serious manner, diplomacy, and dedication to the scientific method earned him respect among his peers at NCI and NIH. This was especially important for an embryonic field that had an uphill struggle to win acceptance as a legitimate discipline. Zubrod could not afford to have his cancer research program seen as a dumping ground for second-class scientists who couldn't make it elsewhere. So he invested heavily in his staff and gave them administrative cover when controversies arose—as they often did.

As one of the NCI clinical associates in the 1950s, I had the good fortune to be involved for a time as this very special collaboration of Zubrod, Freireich, Frei, and their young associates took shape. I feel even more privileged now to pass along their own stories of those years that made NCI the hub of childhood leukemia research.

CHAPTER 7

C. Gordon Zubrod, M.D.

I suppose that there may still be laymen, and even physicians, who are unaware that some cancers can be cured by drugs, but it really is ancient history, almost embarrassingly so for me. The first clinical study that led to the realization that cancer could be so cured started in 1956 and, in the twenty-three years since, at least ten different cancers have been shown to be curable by drugs.

—C. Gordon Zubrod, Myron Karon Memorial Lecture, 1979

If ever there was a maestro who orchestrated the cure of childhood leukemia, it had to be Dr. C. Gordon Zubrod. His protégés, Dr. Frei and Dr. Freireich, and others in the know feel deeply that Gordon has not received sufficient credit for the important role that he played in the fight against leukemia. Credit is not an issue for Dr. Zubrod; indeed, he has spent his career going out of his way to stay out of the limelight, not putting his name on papers that came out of his program at the National Cancer Institute unless he was actively involved in the study, for example, and giving credit to people who actually conducted the experiments. A biographical sketch that appeared some years ago in *Current Biography* made an insightful observation: "Dr. C. Gordon Zubrod is demonstrating that the battle against the disease must be fought in the administrator's office as well as in the laboratory." Not that Dr. Zubrod fought his battles only in the administrator's office: he was an excellent scientist as well. But he had remarkable skills in administrative matters and in organizing clinical investigation in the field of anticancer drugs.

I had the pleasure of working with Dr. Zubrod in the 1950s, as well as with Dr. Frei and Dr. Freireich, but I never really knew about their formative years and early careers until the advent of this book project. Born in Brooklyn in 1914, Gordon Zubrod has one sister—a brother died at the age of seven. Gordon's mother died back in 1921, when she was only in her twenties. During that year the family moved to Baldwin, Long Island, where Gordon obtained his early education. His father was a stockbroker who provided generously for the household. Baldwin was a fishing village on the great South Bay of the Atlantic Ocean, and Gordon spent a great deal of time roaming the inlets and acquiring a love of the sea and an interest in marine biology. He had time for team sports such as baseball, basketball, ice hockey, and individual sports such as swimming, track, and tennis. His athletic activities were limited by a major illness in 1928. Then in the second year of high school, he developed some type of lung infection and probably a viral inflammation of the heart that caused him to miss a year of school. During that time he became interested in medicine and what doctors do. It is of interest that he was befriended by Dr. Sam Hill, the doctor who took care of him, as well as the family doctor, Dr. Painton, who let young Gordon ride around with him on house calls, accompany him to the hospital, and even to "scrub in" on some operations.

Gordon had the notion of becoming a family doctor someday, but first he had to finish his education. He was interested in studying biology, but the boarding school to which his father sent him in 1929, Georgetown Preparatory School, a Jesuit-operated school in Garrett Park, Maryland, was heavily weighted toward the humanities. He thus received a strong background in classics, but only minimal training in science. Nevertheless Gordon felt that the intensive Latin classes helped him to develop good study habits as well as the ability to sort out and analyze problems. In 1932 he entered Holy Cross College as a premedical student, but mainly studied humanities, with just enough science to qualify for medical school. He applied to two medical schools, Columbia and Harvard, and was accepted at both. Columbia cost $530 a year in tuition and Harvard cost only $400, but Gordon liked the people at Columbia and decided to go there. The tuition of that day doesn't seem like a lot of money, but by that time his father, who had prospered in the twenties, had suffered severe losses in the stock market crash of 1929. Gordon paid his way in college by working as a waiter during the day and as a library clerk at night in addition to receiving scholarships. Some of his other jobs included working for the Good Humor Ice Cream Company during the summer and as a night cashier at Presbyterian Hospital while a medical student.

Gordon and Kay were married just five days after he graduated from medical school. By that time he had decided to go into general practice, but he put off his internship in order to earn some money first. (Interns did not receive any salary in those days, and he needed funds in order to finance his internship.) Toward that end he took a position at Central Islip State Hospital, a large psychiatric institution on Long Island. He spent six months at Central Islip, with some six thousand patients, two thousand of whom were Gordon's primary responsibility. He discovered the obvious, that working in a general hospital can be dull; he found out that he was really more interested in internal medicine. To spend his time more productively, he decided to perform complete medical examinations on each of his patients, many of whom had not been examined in their thirty years of residence in the institution, and he detected many previously undiscovered diseases during the course of that experience. For example, he discovered a patient who was a diphtheria carrier, a finding that led to the inoculation of all six thousand of the patients in order to immunize them against the disease.

During that time Kay worked as a medical secretary at Columbia, and she talked with one of Gordon's medical school teachers, Professor Robert Loeb, about Gordon's boredom at Central Islip. Loeb's phenomenal memory was legendary, and he never forgot his former students. (We will hear more about Dr. Loeb later.) Loeb suggested that Gordon should apply for an internship at Columbia. Unfortunately the timing was such that Gordon had just accepted a one-year surgical internship at Jersey City Medical Center, and it was a commitment that he felt bound to fulfill. A person of lesser integrity might have backed out of the Jersey City hospital position, but not Gordon.

It happened that at that time Jersey City had a unique health care system. The famous Mayor Hague had arranged for "free" medical care for everyone in the city—probably the only city in America where free care was available to all. Gordon worked in a twenty-story surgical hospital in Jersey City, and the chief surgeon lived up in the penthouse apartment. At that hospital, Gordon learned a lesson about the need for carefully controlled objective clinical studies and honest statistics in order to avoid bias in clinical trials. The surgeon was interested in gall bladder surgery; whenever the residents would tell him about an "easy gall bladder case" coming to the hospital, he would come down from the penthouse suite and do the operation himself. On the one hand, he could truthfully say that he had performed five hundred consecutive operations without incurring a fatality. That sounded pretty impressive. On the other hand, the residents had to do all the more complicated operations, and so all of the deaths occurred on the residents' service. This biased selection of cases taught Gordon a valuable lesson about comparing results that are not comparable.

After the twelve months in Jersey City were finished, Gordon followed Professor Loeb's advice and entered a two-year internship program at Columbia Presbyterian Hospital in New York. Because of the chaos of war, however, no one really completed a regular program in those days. In March of 1943, Loeb, as head of an advisory committee on clinical research for the Army's Office of Scientific Research and Development (OSRD), recruited Gordon and other young residents in New York hospitals to work on the urgent problem of malaria.

Of all unlikely places, clinical malaria studies were being conducted right there in New York City—at Goldwater Memorial Hospital on Welfare Island (now Roosevelt Island). Gordon was inducted into the army overnight (he went to the Brooklyn Navy Yard for a physical and immunizations) and went to work the next day. He joined a remarkable team of scientists, a "Who's Who" of clinical research of the day, under the leadership of a bright young physician, Dr. James Shannon, who later became director of NIH.

Why New York City as the one place for a major crash research program to study a tropical disease? It had turned out that reliable research on antimalarial treatments in the tropics was impossible. The patients were too apt to be reinfected. But Welfare Island had no mosquitoes that carried the malaria parasite, and there was a ready supply of patients—syphilis patients—to participate in the experiments.

Although it seems absurd at first, the treatment of choice for syphilis in the era before penicillin was to give patients malaria. The rationale, however, was sound: the best way to prevent a horrible brain complication of syphilis (known as general paresis) was to kill the syphilis spirochete, and observation had shown that a high fever that lasted several days could halt the disease in about half the syphilitic patients. Malaria was the best way to induce such a high, long fever. Those were the earliest experiences with formal clinical trials in the United States, and the distinction between research to find a better treatment and the practice of medicine had not been fully recognized. Thus it is doubtful that many of the patients understood the full extent of their participation in the malaria studies, whether or not they benefited. The nature of full disclosure of information and the process of informed consent have evolved over the ensuing five decades.

"When I went to Goldwater Hospital in 1943," Gordon recalls, "I was involved in the most marvelous drug development in our country's history, the malaria program of the OSRD. This was carried out because of the great concern of the Joint Chiefs of Staff about the high casualty rate from malaria among our troops in the South Pacific. We had all kinds of people collaborating on concepts and studies of drug synthesis, screening, toxicity, and running clinical trials to see whether the drugs were effective."

The team of scientists at Goldwater Hospital—perhaps the medical counterpart of the Manhattan Project to make the A-bomb—did a great deal of work on the pharmacology of atabrine. They found a safe way to give this drug, which turned out to be much more effective than quinine at preventing malaria. By taking one pill daily, six days out of every week, servicemen in North Africa, Burma, and the South Pacific stayed free of malaria, certainly a major factor in the Allied forces' ability to wage war there. Out of that drug development program also came chloroquine, for years the best of the antimalarial drugs.

What Gordon learned was that it was possible to bring together the best brains in the country and to have them all work very productively on one difficult subject. The team included basic scientists and clinical scientists, and there was no shortage of money in a national commitment of this type. Normally, the scientific community would be opposed to this type of so-called targeted research, preferring research that is generated by an investigator, according to whatever that person wishes to study. "Well, I believe that both approaches are needed. But in any event, I learned lessons about how to organize clinical trials and those lessons would serve me well later on when I organized a group which intended to cure leukemia, the Acute Leukemia Task Force."

Upon discharge in 1946, Gordon joined the staff of Johns Hopkins University School of Medicine, where he worked in the departments of Pharmacology and Medicine. Over the next seven years he was part of a team of talented scientists doing intensive research on bacterial pneumonia (the disease that had killed his mother) in that most exciting period when the first antibiotics against pneumococcal diseases were being developed. Gordon also served as secretary to a pioneering committee started at

Hopkins by some of the "giants" of American medicine to initiate clinical trials of treatments for infectious diseases. When the Veterans Administration planned its important studies on tuberculosis treatments, they turned to the Hopkins group for guidance. For Gordon, the experience provided invaluable training in ethics, statistics, pharmacology, infectious disease, and the organization of large-scale biomedical research—all crucial to the later fight to cure leukemia.

Following this highly productive period, a midwestern medical school recruited Gordon as associate professor of medicine. It looked like a good opportunity, but Gordon found himself caught in a difficult situation. The chairman wanted to reorganize the institution and make it into a modern Department of Medicine, but the local practitioners and the nurses rebelled and actually refused to refer patients to the hospital. When the administrators tried to break the deadlock, a number of people, including Gordon, lost their jobs. In the meantime some very good house staff had been assembled, including Dr. Emil Frei, the chief resident, whom Gordon would later recruit to the National Cancer Institute, and Dr. Robert Heyssel, later the president of Johns Hopkins Hospital.

When the department folded, Gordon moved to Mount Desert Island Biological Laboratory in Maine, where he did research on the passage of drugs between the blood and the brain of marine animals. The human brain is protected by a screen that effectively filters out the passage of many drugs into the brain. One could not then have predicted that the study of this barrier in animals would someday prove to be a key frontier in the fight against leukemia. Yet ultimately the ill wind that blew Gordon Zubrod to Maine did the search for a leukemia cure a favor.

From Maine, Gordon was recruited to the National Cancer Institute's new Clinical Center in Bethesda, Maryland, by Dr. Shannon, his former colleague in the malaria studies, now scientific director of the Heart Institute. Gordon's job was to develop a cancer chemotherapy program. Gordon began to bring more scientists into the group already gathered there; in 1955 he recruited Dr. Frei and shortly thereafter Dr. Freireich into the leukemia group, followed by a succession of very talented people in other areas of pharmacology and medical research. Soon he was able to attract Dr. Nathaniel Berlin, who later would replace Gordon as clinical director and who was strongly supportive of the leukemia research.

Back in the middle fifties there were very few anticancer drugs available: the nitrogen mustard derivatives, 6-MP, folic acid antagonists such as methotrexate, and a few other drugs that were in the process of study. Gordon advocated a more thorough and systematic approach to the development of anticancer drugs, different from previous approaches that he called a "treasure hunt" for a spectacular cure. In those days, there was a general philosophy that drug treatment of cancer was the last resort—after surgery and radiation had failed—primarily because of the side effects of the available drugs. Gordon and his colleagues set about developing methods for the systematic testing of new compounds, working out new experimental designs in the clinic for anticancer drugs, and setting up programs that tried to predict whether a drug would become useful in the treatment of cancer and leukemia. It was a most challenging task.

Much of the planning was obviously drawn from Gordon's previous experiences in malaria research and in antibiotics. I was curious why he had selected leukemia as the major target, though of course this turned out to be a wise choice. There were several reasons, including the facts that there were at least some active drugs that would affect the disease and there was a relatively quantitative endpoint by which to measure that clinical response. As a practical matter Dr. James Holland was at the National Cancer Institute at the time, and he was particularly interested in the study of leukemia.

Moreover, in NCI's excellent experimental laboratories, Dr. Abraham Goldin had just found that large doses of methotrexate, when given intermittently, gave much better results against mouse leukemia than frequent small doses of the same drug. That was a lead, an indication of a possible path to follow. Gordon and Jim Holland proceeded to design a carefully controlled clinical trial to compare two different ways of giving methotrexate. As Gordon and Jim set out to write the details of the clinical protocol (program), they realized that they needed a better definition of the disease called acute leukemia. There was more to quantitating the disease than just saying whether the patient was well or not. How were they to determine the ways of establishing the *degrees* of sickness and the stages of leukemia relapse when that occurred?

This effort began while Jim Holland was at the National Cancer Institute and continued after he moved to Roswell Park in Buffalo about a month after Gordon arrived in 1954. The program was continued at the National Cancer Institute in 1955 by Tom Frei and J Freireich who, while collaborating with Holland, also began their own studies. In the meantime

99

they were finding it difficult to accumulate sufficient numbers of patients to study, and they had to look to other clinics to join in and pool resources. This became the basis of the first cooperative group to do the clinical studies, the Acute Leukemia Group B. Zubrod, Freireich, and Frei also determined the need for a separate Leukemia Service at the National Cancer Institute, staffed by nurses and doctors who were extremely knowledgeable in the care of patients with this particular illness. This new approach to creating a specialized environment would be widely emulated by other institutions in the future.

In another organizational step that Gordon valued, physicians from the five major cancer centers in the country began to meet every year and put on demonstrations for each other. At the Boston meeting hosted by Dr. Farber in 1955, Gordon talked about the cooperative group formed between the National Cancer Institute and Holland's team at Roswell Park and asked whether others wanted to join. They were satisfied with their programs at Harvard and at Memorial Sloan-Kettering in New York, however, and decided not to participate. The National Cancer Institute had not yet become the center of leukemia research for the world.

It was at the 1955 Boston meeting that the various investigators began to talk about the need for more information about leukemia and for a definition of a response to treatment so that the results at one institution could be compared with those at another. Without common definitions and a uniform system of reporting, cooperative studies were not really possible. Gordon recalls that, at the end of one meeting, several of them went off to talk about the bone marrow test as a quantitative measure of the number of leukemic cells present, and whether it might be used to define what was meant by a partial and a complete remission (response). Up to then, only blood counts and the number of leukemic cells in the blood had been used as the endpoint to measure a remission. But, as seems so obvious to us now, and as they learned from their studies, the bone marrow has in it a great deal more information than such simple measures. Freireich, who was trained as a hematologist, and Frei followed up the conversation by developing the bone marrow examination as an endpoint. All of the groups began to use this as an index soon thereafter, a major technical advance.

Gordon Zubrod thus set the stage for the systematic study of the various manifestations of leukemia and for concentration on the complications of the disease and its treatment. Furthermore, because of his own previous interest in infectious disease and because infections in patients with leukemia were a major problem, he and the group were most anxious to describe the different types of infections accurately and to determine how often they occurred.

As I have noted, at the National Cancer Institute at that time there was not only the senior staff but also a series of bright young doctors who had joined the Public Health Service and who were assigned to rotate through the services over a period of two years. (Some envious colleagues called us the Yellow Berets.) Very often these clinical associates had better or more extensive clinical training than the staff researchers who supervised them, some of whom had only one year of internship after medical school. Particularly important in working with J Freireich and Tom Frei on the problem of characterizing infections were the clinical associates Doctors Dane Boggs, Claude Forkner, Jr., Dick Fritz, Richard Shaw, Richard Silver, and, later on, Gerald Bodey and Evan Hersh.

It turned out that the ability to recognize the types of bacterial and fungus infections and to diagnose them early, and to understand the relationship between the susceptibility to infection and the level of white blood cells, made it possible to develop new methods to prevent and treat these infections. This was extremely important in preventing the death of patients before they could even have time to achieve a remission in leukemia from the drug treatment.

There were similar problems related to the management of hemorrhage and the risk of early death from low platelet counts and bleeding into the brain. These problems were also to be worked out at the National Cancer Institute. The studies would result in the classic work on the importance of platelets, which would completely surprise the hematology community. But the world did not change easily. The bright young investigators were up against the established ideas of the day. And it was Dr. Zubrod who supported their efforts.

Many people have speculated about how the idea that it might be possible to *cure* leukemia actually originated. The insight may have come in 1961, at about the time when Gordon was hospitalized for severe gastrointestinal bleeding. At that juncture, the director of the National Cancer Institute was Dr. Kenneth Endicott, and he wanted Gordon to become his new scientific director. Gordon first turned it down, then later agreed to take the job. But in his discussions with Endicott he explained that there were five drugs, each of which had activity against leukemia, and that it was time to form an interdisciplinary group, a thinking-and-planning committee, the purpose of which would be to use these drugs with the intention to cure leukemia. This visionary effort, later called the Acute Leukemia Task Force, would be separate from the cooperative group, though that group would be represented on the task force and would implement any clinical trials that were suggested.

They wanted to leap forward, but careful planning would be required. Endicott proposed that they go and visit IBM and study its task force methods. He and Gordon spent some days with IBM and were attracted to the approach of industry. It seems that when IBM got onto a hot lead, it would take four or five scientists off other projects and put them together to work at the problem until they could determine whether or not they had something. This was a good idea for large industry, but it wasn't suitable for working with leukemia scientists because the top experts were located in different institutions. A unifying mechanism for a strike force of that kind was needed. Gordon visited the key political leaders in the cancer field, who at that time were Dr. Isadore Ravdin at the University of Pennsylvania and Dr. Sidney Farber, and they gave the idea their blessing. Those influential doctors weren't necessary to do the work, but once they approved of the idea the young people would sign on. So now the National Cancer Institute had the money and the political clout to develop a task force of the best investigators, and this it did under the leadership of Gordon Zubrod.

The group itself eventually met about once a month. In this way Gordon was also able to recruit investigators at other institutions peripheral to Washington and Bethesda to consider his problems, and he had many. For example, there was the relationship of the task force to the Cancer Chemotherapy National Service Center (CCNSC), which was located on the campus of the National Institutes of Health. The group was investigating the effects of some 30,000 compounds a year on experimental tumors in mice, but did not include sufficient senior scientists to study its results. This program was generating huge amounts of data that few experts even reviewed. It was a mammoth undertaking and often rather mindless, or so it seemed to me.

The task force arranged to look at the data by breaking it out into different categories—one dealing with the screening data in which they looked at drugs that had inhibitory activity against certain types of mouse tumors. The category was then further broken down by having a separate group of scientists look at the toxicity to examine the different types of side effects of the chemicals, and so forth. Gordon wanted to know what was going on in other laboratories, as well. He brought in their best investigators to contribute their findings to those of the task force.

When you put bright people together, unexpected and productive things can happen: some of them can be quite humorous. It was at about this time that the question of whether viruses caused leukemia was generating great excitement. Dr. Jack Dalton, an excellent virologist at the National Cancer Institute, had developed a new method of staining viruses, and he thought he was finding virus particles in the blood of many patients who had leukemia. This finding was so remarkable that the topic was included in a task force meeting and the data were presented to the group. Dr. Dalton was also studying a type of lymphoma in cattle, and he described what he thought were identical virus particles in the milk of cows. Amazed to learn about this, several people went rushing down to the Department of Agriculture, which became very upset upon hearing the news. They asked that the scientific data not be published right away, but that the findings be studied further. Otherwise, they said, it would cause a panic in the vital dairy industry, not to mention in the mothers of America! The next day the National Cancer Institute received ten million dollars from Agriculture with which to pursue viral research as rapidly as possible.

Dr. Zubrod secured the help of an experienced virologist at NCI, Dr. Ray Bryan, and together they drew up a program for virus research in leukemia. This was the beginning of what was to become a huge program. Other viral experts were brought in to serve as an advisory committee, including two Nobel laureates, Dick Shope and Wendell Stanley. They looked at all of the data and advised the director that the National Cancer Institute scientists were onto something real and important, even though, as it turned out, Dalton's particles were not viruses at all, but rather an artifact. There were no true virus particles in blood and milk, just submicroscopic particles induced by the new staining method: an honest but embarrassing error for many excellent scientists. It is fascinating to reflect that the driving force—and the money—that started the important virus program at the National Cancer Institute was really attributable to an artifact, a matter that has not been discussed publicly or is even recognized by the broad community of researchers. Later the program did become tremendously productive. The polio program had just been completed, and many first-rate virologists were looking for new worlds to conquer.

Another important product of the work of the task force was the recognition that a particular kind of mouse leukemia, the so-called L_{1210}, discovered by an NCI scientist, Dr. Lloyd Law, was the very best animal model with which to work out drug schedules. It was not only useful in looking for antileukemic activity of drugs, but, just as important, it was a useful predictor of how to utilize those drugs. Doctors Howard Skipper at Southern Research Institute and Abe Goldin at NCI pioneered the use of this model. Skipper and his associates demonstrated conclusively that one had to kill off the last remaining leukemic cell in order to cure mice that had this leukemia. In order to do that, one had to go on treating the animals long after the clinical evidence of the disease had disappeared. In other words, despite the fact that mice were apparently in remission, they were still harboring leukemic cells that would eventually result in a relapse unless the treatment was continued sufficiently to kill all of the cells.

This is where scientists were with their patients who were in remission, knowing that the disease had apparently disappeared and yet also knowing all the while that there still had to be leukemic cells present. With this knowledge, obviously, the decision to stop or not to stop treatment was fraught with all kinds of emotional stress. The work of Skipper and his colleagues was critical in thinking about subsequent strategies for treating patients who were in remission. Their work with mouse leukemia would prove to be useful to Frei and to the other cooperative groups led by Burchenal and others in designing new types of chemotherapy approaches. The usual unwritten scientific practice was for individual institutions to follow up the scientific leads garnered from studies on animals and to do pilot studies on a limited number of patients. Then larger cooperative groups would come along to study greater numbers of patients to exploit the new idea and put it to rigorous scientific test. That was the plan.

You might wonder how one translates the dosage of a drug from a mouse to a human. In other words, if you work out a dosage schedule (that is, the dose, frequency, and route of administration), what does that mean for treating a four-year-old child or an overweight fifty-year-old adult? The discovery of how to set different doses for humans was another dividend that came from the Acute Leukemia Task Force, specifically from a toxicity group consisting of Skipper, David Rall, Freireich, and Leon Schmidt. The conversion of dosages from animals to humans had previously been done according to a formula based on the weight of the animal, and this was also utilized in translating the dosage from an adult to a child. However, this group systematically worked out that it was far preferable to calculate drug dosage on the basis of the body surface area as the unit of measure. If you did that, you could directly transfer the relevance of toxicity data from animals to humans according to a proportionality formula. This was a milestone in drug development not only in cancer but with other drugs and other diseases as well. The system doesn't work equally well for all drugs, but it was particularly useful in studies of childhood leukemia. Don Pinkel, for one, made good use of this information in treating his patients. It seems like a trivial point, but to be able to predict the dosage of drugs that may cause toxicity is a very important factor in providing safety to a child who is under treatment with a new drug.

Another scientific milestone in the battle against leukemia came with the discovery of the usefulness of the drug vincristine. This drug, a natural substance extracted from the ubiquitous periwinkle plant, was highly active in childhood leukemia. This whole opportunity might have been missed had it not been for the administrative efforts of Tom Frei and Gordon Zubrod. Eli Lilly, the company making vincristine, had given it out for research study at four or five institutions, but none had seen much activity with it except Frei's team at the National Cancer Institute. (J Freirich describes this work in more detail in his chapter.) Because of the failure at the other institutions, the Lilly Company thought that it wasn't worthwhile to keep on producing the drug. It planned to shelve the project and develop only vinblastine, another periwinkle alkaloid substance. But Gordon and Tom Frei flew out to Lilly's corporate headquarters in Indianapolis to present the new data they had obtained and to plead for vincristine to continue to be made available for research study. That personal visit was sufficient to prompt the firm to continue making the drug. Eventually, the combined use of steroids and vincristine made a huge difference in the remission rate of childhood acute leukemia, and would prove to have been an extraordinarily important step.

During the course of carefully designed scientific studies, one hopes to achieve the specific aims of the study by the analysis of meticulously collected data, and this was being done at NCI. Then there is always the opportunity of coming across a surprising finding under the heading of serendipity. As we have seen, serendipity, or luck, comes to those with prepared minds, and there are many such instances in the leukemia story. But there is still another facet of success that may commonly be called a "fluke" or a statistically unlikely event. Gordon recalls one of these quite vividly from the early days of the National Cancer Institute program.

The staff admitted a little girl who was terminally ill and who, it appeared, would surely die within just a matter of days. She was so sick that they only gave her steroids in the form of prednisone, hoping that she would improve enough so that she could be treated with more standard types of chemotherapy. But after two weeks she had achieved a complete remission, and the doctors decided to wait to treat her further until she relapsed at a later date. Ten years later she was still in a complete remission, and Gordon happened to see her picture in the newspaper as a basketball player for her school. "At that point we went back to review her original blood slides with the blood specialist at the National Cancer Institute, who was an expert in leukemia. He reviewed the slides and said that although he had originally called it leukemia, it probably wasn't that because the patient had survived so long!" This illustrates the point that doctors, even super experts, had preconceived ideas about the incurability of leukemia. That kind of thinking was an important barrier to be surmounted in devising strategies to cure the disease.

One of the great things that Zubrod did was to visualize NCI, including its Clinical Center, as a place where one could have a great range and depth of scientists to do things that could not be done in community hospitals. "Private doctors don't like to make their patients too sick and so they don't treat them aggressively enough to give them the opportunity for a cure, at least until others have done it first and shown how to go about doing it. The other aspect of a center is that there are experts in various different disciplines, where you can really get a critical mass of people together to look at a single problem from different scientific points of view. It is like a college without walls. This is difficult to do in medical schools as well, where there is a good deal of protection of the academic turf. I have been very fortunate to have had such opportunities in the case of malaria research during World War II and again in the leukemia program at NCI. All kinds of research are necessary, both basic and clinical. Too often there are arguments about the type of research that is preferable, but I like to think of the words of Pasteur, quoted by René Vallery-Radot in his 1927 biography: 'There does not exist a category of science to which one can give the name applied science. There are science and the applications of science, bound together as the fruit to the tree which bears it.' "

CHAPTER 8

Emil J Freireich, M.D.

It ain't bragging if you really done it.
—Dizzy Dean

I've known Emil J Freireich since the mid-1950s, when we were both young medical researchers at the National Cancer Institute. He was brash, cocky, full of dreams, and given to hyperbole. To the NCI fellows—the young doctors primarily responsible for taking care of the children on NCI's leukemia ward—J's visits were a mixed blessing. During bleak days on the ward, his enthusiasm for his latest notion for treating the children was refreshing *and* infuriating. We respected his leadership, envied his self-confidence and single-mindedness of purpose, and, more than once, mocked his "crazy ideas."

Over the ensuing years he has mellowed, but he is still as controversial as ever. Fortunately, he thrives on controversy. At times his argumentativeness and lack of political skill have cost him offices and honors in oncology circles, but he has never been one to compromise. It has always been a short trip between the top of his mind and the tip of his tongue, and in some ways the interaction between his personality and the application of science has been both his greatest asset and his greatest liability. He is certainly one of a kind, and he is easier to understand if we hear some of his story in his own voice.

''I am different from most other, more sophisticated guys. I was born in 1927 of Hungarian immigrant parents and I am a child of the post–World War I era. My father owned a restaurant during the gay twenties but lost everything to the Depression. He died shortly thereafter of a mysterious illness—possibly suicide. I was only two years old at the time. My mother was poor and had to do piecework to support herself, my sister, and me. We lived in a Chicago ghetto—it was like a third world nation. All that mattered to us was food, clothing, shelter, and safety from the ghetto gangs. We struggled to survive, and it colors the way I think.

"By the age of eight or nine, I knew only one male who had any human quality: a Jewish general practitioner by the name of Dr. Rosenbloom. He liked what he was doing even though he didn't get paid. When anyone got sick, Dr. Rosenbloom came around. He had no medicines to speak of; he was just a caring and dignified person. Later, when I became a 'famous' cancer doctor, I went back to that area in Chicago, and you know, he was doing the same thing. He probably died doing the same thing. He loved everybody, and I always wanted to be like that."

If someone had told J's mother that her son would someday become a successful cancer researcher, she wouldn't have known what he was talking about. She could barely speak English, let alone help him with schoolwork. Nonetheless, his academic performance during elementary and high school was very good. Tuley High School (now called Roberto Clemente High School) was "simply an exercise in discipline, just a way to keep you off the streets." But J had a physics teacher who took pride in identifying bright young students. One day the teacher asked him, "Freireich, would you like to go to college?"

J said, "College, how do you do that?"

The teacher told him, "They have this state school that pays your tuition; it's called the University of Illinois."

"That sounds nice. How do I afford it and how do I get there?"

J convinced his mother that he should continue his education. His wish to become a doctor did the trick. She took him to a charitable Christian Scientist friend, who patted his head and asked, "How much do you need?" Her gift of $25 made college possible for J. He used $6 of the $25 for a railroad ticket to Urbana-Champaign, his first trip away from home. He was sixteen at the time.

"Even though I had not preregistered and the university had no record of my high school performance, they were kind enough to allow me to register tentatively for the premedical program. Registration cost another $13. The registrar advised me to get a job at a sorority, where I served meals, bussed dishes, and mopped the floor for $3 a week plus meals. In the second semester I was able to get a scholarship. I really wasn't that different from the other kids attending this land-grant college. They all came from families without education or means."

In the spring of 1945, J had his eighteenth birthday and received his draft notice. By then he had completed one and a half years of undergraduate work and needed only to complete that semester in order to meet the requirements for admission to medical school. Much to his disgust, the enthusiastic young patriot was rejected by the draft board doctor on flimsy grounds. J finished up at the University of Illinois.

"I went back to Chicago, moved in with my mother, and took the elevated train to the University of Illinois College of Medicine.

"I did very well in medical school—I was not ambitious, but I learned fast. I was sixth among the two hundred students in the first-year class and graduated at about that same rank in 1949. During one of my first-year classes a teacher asked me if I had cheated, because my grades were so high. I was so offended that I never spoke to him again."

For his internship, J wanted to study in the Chicago area and was lucky enough to be accepted by his first choice, the Cook County Hospital.

"My career of being an unpleasant person began during my first month as an intern at Cook County. Cook County Hospital—a huge public facility—was a remarkably unpleasant place to practice. For example, within a period of one week I would guess that I admitted thirty-five patients with congestive heart failure, and yet I didn't know how to treat the disease.

"The story of Ward 55 sums up what that place was like for me and the patients. After I'd worked up an interesting patient who was terribly ill with a hematologic condition, I came back to the ward one day and couldn't find the patient. I learned that the head nurse had assigned the patient to a room off to the side of the ward. Walking into that room, I became nauseated and almost vomited. There were twenty beds packed so closely together that you couldn't walk between them. Patients who were not expected to live were placed in those beds and left there without food, water, or changes of clothing. No one survived, they just died in their feces and urine, and were carted out of the room. Then the nurse looked for the next suitable candidate. I was furious and told the nurse that this couldn't continue. Her reply was that she'd been there for many years and that I was new, and that's the way the ward was run. I complained to the hospital director, who told me that the head nurse was in charge. If I didn't like it, I could leave. However, he reminded me that, if

I did leave, I would be breaking my contract. I tried to buck the system, but the best I could do was to be transferred to another ward.

"As I rotated through the various services—Medicine, Surgery, all the other brands of medicine—my reputation as a troublemaker preceded me. I was constantly back in the hospital director's office, like a little child being sent to the principal. At last, the director, as tired of me as I was of the hospital, offered to release me from my contract after one and a half years instead of two, if I could find someone to take over the remainder of my internship. I found a medical student to replace me and went across the street to work as a resident on the medical service of Dr. S. Howard Armstrong of Rush Presbyterian Hospital."

The move out of Cook County Hospital was a lucky break for J. At that point, he had no idea what a career in research was all about. Relatively few medical schools were then academically oriented; they were content to turn out practicing physicians. J had no one to show him what a medical researcher in academic medicine did.

"When I left the Cook County Hospital and walked into Presbyterian, I was like a starving man who had walked into a supermarket. I had thought the world of medicine had been at Cook County Hospital, but now I was surrounded by intellectual giants. This new world was a revelation to me.

"First of all, there was Dr. Armstrong, a sophisticated and elegant man who seemed to know everything about medicine. He had come to Chicago from Harvard as a disciple of the famous Dr. Soma Weiss, the father of clinical investigation in this country. Around 1950 Dr. Armstrong became chairman of medicine at Rush Presbyterian Hospital. He employed the teaching methods he'd learned in Boston, emphasizing the training of residents and students and teaching about research and physiology. Everyone was excited to be around him. He had worked with Dr. E. J. Cohen developing albumin, which had been so important as a plasma substitute during the war. He was full of ideas. Even as a student at Cook County Hospital I had gone to attend some of his conferences at Presbyterian Hospital and I couldn't believe anyone was that smart—he knew everything and I used to sit in awe of him.

"Dr. Armstrong cut quite a dashing figure in Chicago—he was a very rich bachelor, had a boat, and made out with the women. However, the hospital authorities couldn't stand him. For one thing, the house staff was loyal to Armstrong and paid no attention to the other physicians on the staff, whose training was much inferior. For another, he scandalized the hospital. You see, rich white people went to Presbyterian for their medical care, and there was the chairman of medicine, always in the paper in connection with various unseemly doings! He died young of hepatitis and probably cirrhosis of the liver.

"Because he was so rich, he didn't give a damn about what the hospital administration thought. What he really cared about was the house staff, the interns and residents. There was nothing he wanted to do more than to be a doctor and teach students, meet with the house staff, make rounds, do research. He was so committed to work that his social activities were bacchanalian—boom and all of a sudden have an orgy and that's it and then back to work, twenty-four hours a day. Even in the middle of the night he'd stop by and see what he could do to assist with patient calls and to teach.

"Howie represented the new medicine from Boston, but there were some other good guys from the old Rush Medical College Clinic. Dr. Woodyatt impressed me the most. He became world famous in the 1930s for recognizing that, if you limit sugar intake and switch the diabetic patient to dietary protein, the carbohydrate metabolism improved. That started the whole dietetic management of diabetes. Woodyatt had been intimately involved in the discovery of insulin. The race to discover insulin was like breaking the genetic code—everybody knew what had to be done, you just had to break it. He impressed us with the excitement and the importance of discovery in research. He made us realize that you have to get some feeling for the value of discovery, because you're surely not going to get paid for it, you're not going to get a prize for it, you may not even be recognized for it: it's just a pleasure to be part of the process of discovery. That's what you got from people like Armstrong and Woodyatt.

"One time I said to Dr. Woodyatt, 'Why didn't you discover insulin, since you were the one who had the clinic and all the resources? After all, Banting and Best, who got the credit for discovering insulin, were just a couple of wet-behind-the-ear guys who were struggling in a fellowship or something, and they weren't anybody compared to you at that time—why didn't you succeed?' 'Well,' he replied, 'if the truth be known, we did succeed.' Woodyatt *had* isolated something from the islets of the pancreas that lowered the blood sugar in diabetic patients, but he wasn't satisfied with the quality of the response. In other words, he had gained some control of the metabolic abnormalities of diabetics, but it wasn't a complete control of sugar levels because they had a very crude product that had insulin (though, of course they didn't call it insulin) in it; they were certain of that. And then Banting and Best made their claim and all of the competing laboratory people, including Woodyatt, ran to Toronto to watch how they'd made it to see if it could be confirmed. He saw how Banting and Best did it in their lab, and he saw the answer to some of the problems that he'd been having. He had not known about one specific and crucial step that Banting and Best had discovered. When he learned that from them, he said, 'Goddamn it, why didn't I think of that?' And he went home and did it and sure enough they were right.

"Three months later he got a call from either Banting or Best saying that their own last batch of insulin didn't work, and was his working and he said, 'Oh yes, perfectly,' so then Banting and Best came to Chicago to see what *they* were doing wrong. It's not important how it all came out. What was important was the involvement in this struggle to discover a life-saving substance, insulin. They weren't competing, there was fame and glory and the Nobel Prize of course, but the real gut, the real competition, was to solve the problem of treating diabetes. Woodyatt wanted his patients to get insulin so they'd get better. And he would get so excited when he told these stories. Once they had insulin, God, it was incredible to think of all the people who used to die of diabetic acidosis; and now they were coming out of it and getting well and they were saving all of the kids who had been dying. He was a giant among investigators, he cared about his patients and about his research. And when you said to him, 'Banting and Best got all the credit and you didn't get any,' he'd answer, 'Well, I got the credit of taking care of patients and I'm very pleased with what I did.' He was a magnificent man.

"Another doctor I admired was Dr. J. B. Herrick, for his pioneering research in the description of myocardial infarction [heart attack] and of the pain of angina pectoris [chest pain due to narrowing of coronary arteries]. As a medical student Herrick had also described sickle-cell anemia. At the time, of course, he wasn't a hematologist and he had almost no tools; he just had his clinical senses. Just to see a man who discovered something as important as that was impressive to me. It was phenomenal to think of the impact of myocardial infarction in our modern culture and to think that, until this guy—who was alive and making rounds with me— figured it out, no one even knew what people were dying of.

"So all of that converted me from a Cook County Hospital atmosphere where you just put on Band-Aids and Scotch tape, to an academic environment where these guys had all discovered things. In medical school I had met only one professor who convinced me that there was anything more to medicine than what the professors taught. Most of the medical school teaching in those days was pretty much by rote; you only had to know the standard material that was in the medical textbooks.

"It was very different at Rush Presbyterian. When I went to Presbyterian, I tried to be like Howie, and I was a brilliant resident. I was very idealistic. I really wanted to help people who were sick and I was reputed to be a very hard-nosed resident with the house staff. But a lot of the interns that worked with me are still my friends. I worked very hard and lived in the hospital. We were a house staff that worked twenty-four hours a day, seven days a week. I'd call it total immersion, but I was totally uneducated, so I wasn't arrogant. All of the staff thought I was a very bright serious student, because I made rounds with all of the attendings [senior physicians] and watched all of the patients and I was compulsive about learning everything.

"Sometimes, though, I would have a run-in with some of the faculty or the older, private doctors who would say, 'Do this,' and I'd look at the x-ray and I'd look at the patient and I'd say, 'I'm sorry, but that's not the right thing to do and I want to give him digitalis (or whatever), and I'm certain I am right and I have the references to prove it.' Then the guy would say, 'Shut your f—— face and do what I say.' And then we'd have a fight and I'd be in big trouble. I couldn't (and still can't) operate in an environment where I had to do what I didn't think was right. I knew I didn't know everything, but I did know something. If people made me do something just because they said so, I couldn't accept that. Howie Armstrong always protected the house staff, so I never had a serious controversy while he was there. But when he got fired, I didn't last five minutes!

"I met with him then privately and said, 'Dr. Armstrong, when you're gone and the teaching service is disbanded, I'm not going to learn anything.' He said, 'Well, quite frankly, Freireich, I'd quit and go to Boston if I were you. You've got to learn some high-powered medicine.' So I went from his office to the office of the hospital administrator, and said, 'I know I have a contract with Presbyterian Hospital, but, to be totally honest with you, I came here because of the teaching service and because of Dr. Armstrong. Now that's been dissolved, I don't honestly believe I'll learn anything more in medicine here. So if you would accept it, I will resign.' In fact, as soon as Howie said, 'Go to Boston,' I packed up my old car, kissed my girlfriend Deanie (later my wife) good-bye, and drove off with my letters of recommendation. I had never been outside the state."

Armstrong's recommendation enabled this huge, rough-cut young doctor to get a job with Dr. Joe Ross at Massachusetts Memorial Hospital in Boston. Ross, an old-style hematology investigator, worked at an outstanding clinical research program run by the famous Dr. Chester Keefer. At that time, J was unaware that Dr. Keefer had not only established the first clinical research center in the United States but also had played a key role in penicillin research in this country. Keefer was a reserved, private person, with a brilliant mind and a photographic memory.

Of Keefer, J recollected: "He was quite a doctor and far, far, far above us. When Dr. Keefer came onto the ward, people just trembled with awe. You didn't fail to comb your hair or dare wear your tie crooked around him. Everyone had a white coat and the patients' sheets all had to be clean. He was a meticulous, compulsive, obsessive physician par excellence, and his social life and his teaching were the same. His third-year student rounds were famous. It was his philosophy that you study on a patient carefully, not a hundred patients sloppily like at the Cook County Hospital. So each student had to present a case to Dr. Keefer once, and all of the house staff and fellows would come, because these occasions were intellectual tours de force.

"Once a medical student presented a patient who had the disease called lupus erythematosus [LE]: Keefer asked the student if he knew about the new LE test to diagnose lupus. That LE blood test had just been published by Hargraves of the Mayo Clinic a few months before this case was presented. Keefer gave him the citation to look up in the Mayo Clinic *Proceedings*. Then Keefer perused the room to see if anyone else was familiar with that article and he looked at me and said, 'Freireich, would you tell this student how to do an LE test?' I said, 'Yes sir,' because I used to do them for the laboratories, and I described this rather complicated test for the student on rounds. Well, for a Chicago hick that was impressive. Keefer said, 'I think you're right; that is the Boston system.' "

The haphazard medical education of J Freireich began to take a more rigorous turn. Still, he had had no direct experience in medical research. That would begin with his boss, Dr. Ross, who was the first scientist in the world to give radioactive iron, first to animals and then to people, in order to measure the life span of red blood cells and to study the metabolism of the oxygen-carrying pigment, hemoglobin.

Ross was an excellent experimentalist, and J credits him in many ways for being responsible for his going into research. Ross assigned him after only two days in Boston to work on an experiment on red blood cells at the Harvard Medical School with Dr. Cliff Barger. J worked endlessly on this project, pipetting blood and solutions, measuring radioactivity with the Geiger counter, measuring radioactive solutions, and injecting radioisotopes into dogs at four o'clock in the morning in order to measure their blood volumes. Ross did his own share of these tasks, and by the age of forty he had developed cataracts in his eyes—undoubtedly from radiation exposure.

This group was studying the factors that affected the life span of the red blood cell. Under some conditions, the cells were destroyed rapidly, causing a condition called hemolytic anemia. But the methods for quantitating this were just being developed in this laboratory. To diagnose the extent of the condition the researchers decided to quantitate the breakdown products of hemoglobin metabolism in the urine and the stool as an indirect measure of how much hemoglobin had been destroyed from the red blood cells. Adapting a technique worked out by Dr. Cecil Watson of Minnesota, Ross, Barger, and their colleagues developed new ways to measure hemoglobin. The amount of bile pigments in the urine and the stool would tell them indirectly how many red blood cells were being destroyed and how fast.

"I had to get all of Watson's papers out of the library and line up the reagents. You set them up like you're going to make steak tartare: you get a cookbook—the publications—and you read the directions. First, you have to go get a stool. So you go and collect crap in a jar for the four-day stool samples. If you've never stood in front of a four-day stool sample, you can't imagine what it's like, especially in a hot, non–air-conditioned room. The directions were simple. You literally pour it into another container, you had to scrape the shit off the bottom and the sides, and add a little water to it, then put in some more solvents like ether to extract the bile pigments, and so forth. Then I'd write the results in a notebook. No one in the lab had ever experienced such awful smells before, but it didn't bother me because I was so excited to be doing anything that was original. It was horrible, but I knew it was important. I *needed* to quantitate those bile pigments, and who in the hell was going to do it for me? I couldn't get the technician to do it, so I did it myself. So, *I'd* be the one who could say, 'God, look at this patient, he's got a high urobilogen, and that means he's hemolyzing [destroying his red blood cells].' That's the good thing about the laboratory we were working in: everybody worked the same way. There was no guy sitting in an office on the top floor who said, 'Do this.' Ours was the first lab to do it and I became the immediate authority on the subject.

"Then we learned about the primary importance of iron metabolism in patients who had anemia in association with inflammatory disorders, such as rheumatoid arthritis. I discovered that the main expert in hematology in the world, Dr. Max Wintrobe, was wrong: his theory was that low serum iron was the main cause of this form of anemia. We demonstrated that the real problem was in the transfer of the iron from the tissues into the red blood cells that were being made in the bone marrow. When I first showed the data to Ross, he didn't believe it. In fact, when we first wrote up the paper, the *Journal of Clinical Investigation* turned it down after it was reviewed. Dr. Ross confronted the editor, who then decided to publish the data. And so my first paper was in the very prestigious *Journal of Clinical Investigation*, and it was on a terrific scientific advance.

"I was working twenty hours a day as a research fellow and I was in love with Deanie. Those were the best years of my life. Then in 1954 the military decided to draft all of the doctors, lest it lose them because of a change in the draft laws. When Dr. Keefer heard I was to be drafted late in 1954, he called me in. Well, I've never been so frightened in my life, because I didn't know what he wanted to see me about. But he said that he understood that I'd been drafted and that I was pretty good. He asked me if I'd ever heard of the National Institutes of Health.

" 'No, sir.'

" 'Well,' he said, 'you can go to the NIH and serve your country there.'

"I had wanted to serve my country in a direct way, for I was still a patriotic young man, but he persuaded me that the National Institutes of Health would be a good place for my career."

The opportunity of a lifetime, as it turned out to be, came out of that conversation with Dr. Keefer. The National Institutes of Health had recently been established, and the Clinical Center for research on patients had only opened in 1953, in the Washington, D.C., suburb, Bethesda. Dr. Keefer had been appointed an assistant secretary for health, education, and welfare and commuted between Boston and Washington regularly. He simply picked up a red phone in his Boston hospital office that gave him a direct line to Washington, spelled out the name of Freireich to an associate there, and told him to fix up a commission in the U.S. Public Health Service. After that, things moved fast.

J went home to tell Deanie that he had to be in Washington in the morning. He would take the overnight bus so he could be in Bethesda by 8:00 A.M. for interviews with the National Institutes for the study of the heart, arthritis, and cancer.

The Arthritis Institute already had a lot of hematologists, and the Heart Group didn't seem interested in J. He finally saw Dr. Gordon Zubrod of the National Cancer Institute. Zubrod thought that NCI needed someone to work on leukemia and asked J if he knew anything about it. Because his former boss, Dr. Ross, had not been interested in leukemia, J had taken care of all of the leukemia cases at the Boston hospital. He was also aware of the work of Dr. Farber with the folate antagonists. When J demonstrated his knowledge to Dr. Zubrod, he was hired on the spot.

J returned to Boston that night and stayed just long enough to pick up his laboratory notebooks, load up his car, and move his young family to Bethesda. He had married Haroldine (Deanie) Lee Cunningham the year before. Deanie had been the head nurse in the outpatient clinic at Rush Presbyterian. She had come out from Chicago to visit J—and stayed to marry him.

"I vividly recall that move. The car had to transport not only all of our belongings but also our nine-month-old infant daughter, my four-months-pregnant wife, and myself. It was hot in Washington and hot on the way down in the car. We drove right up to the front door of the NIH Clinical Center, and Deanie and the baby stayed in the car while I reported for active duty. I was told, 'There's your office, you can go to work,' but I said, 'My wife is still sitting out in the car.' We managed to find a room, and we were pretty well settled within the month.

"A very curious thing happened when I walked down the twelfth floor corridor of the clinical center to find my office: I saw the name Dr. Emil Frei on a door that I thought was my office. My first thought, of course, was, 'Isn't this typical of the government, they even misspelled my name.' When I entered the office, I found this tall, thin young man who identified himself as Emil Frei. We quickly realized that we were both recently hired

118

by Dr. Zubrod and were working with the same group. The striking similarity of our names was quite a coincidence. Actually, my office was directly next door to his. Dr. Frei and I worked closely together not only as colleagues but as personal friends for the next seventeen years. But the confusion about our names continues to this day. Imagine the odds against a Dr. Emil Frei and a Dr. Emil Freireich working together!

"The names have always put us in the posture of representing each other. I've been invited to give talks and meetings where people say things like, 'Oh you wrote that great book, *Cancer Medicine,*' and I have to reply, 'No, that's the other guy.' When I was awarded the Karnofsky Prize, Dr. Joe Burchenal introduced me and gave me the medal. He read the back of it and said, 'This is given to Emil "Tom" Freireich.' I also get called by the name 'Emil J Freireich III' all the time. And of course the same thing happens to Tom. He'll be introduced as Emil J Frei III, or J Frei. Occasionally I get a letter that is clearly intended for him, and we receive many phone calls that belong to each other. There was a period of time when most people thought there was only one person. You see, we didn't always publish as coauthors on the same papers, and there were many publications where there was only one of us as an author on the paper. There were people who used to believe that there was only one person and that we'd had a misspelling problem."

Emil Frei III had been nicknamed Tom when he was still a small child, to distinguish him from his father and grandfather in the same house. Emil J Freireich had picked up his nickname as an adult. He did not even know about the middle J in his name until he was eighteen and had to get a copy of his birth certificate for the Selective Service. "What's this J in the middle of my name?" he asked his mother. "Oh," she said, "that's easy to understand. You see, they write your name as Freireich, Emil. I explained to the woman that I wanted to name you after my grandfather, so she told me that you were to be Emil Freireich, Junior" So his mother simply put in the "J" for junior, and the name was transcribed as Emil J Freireich.

Before Freireich got married, Deanie told him that the name Emil didn't appeal to her. "When Deanie heard the story about my birth certificate and that my name was really Emil J Freireich, she said, 'Well, that's it, we'll just call you J.' So from that point on my middle initial became my name and I accepted the acronym because I didn't want to be a junior. My middle name is simply the letter J without a period after it, like Harry S Truman. Of course when I publish papers I write my name Emil J and they always want to put a period after it. I take the period out of the galley proofs and they put it back in. About 80 percent of my publications have a period after the letter J. So I've been called J for years and no one calls me Emil: my kids don't even know me by that name. When I met Emil Frei for the first time, I said, 'That's ridiculous, that's my name.' He said, 'You can just call me Tom,' and I told him, 'For sure don't call me Emil, my name's J, or my wife will throw you out of our house!' "

Was it just the accidental meeting of J Freireich with Gordon Zubrod that led to the tremendous burst of productivity in leukemia research? Nothing in J's previous professional life suggested that he would have a special interest in leukemia. However, a personal experience may have been a strong subconscious motivation: while he was in medical school his life was deeply touched by a young woman who died of leukemia.

"I finished high school at the age of sixteen—I was still prepubescent, short, and obese. So I wasn't much at athletics and I wasn't a big hit with either the girls or the boys. I did make a close friendship with Leonard Reich, who was a little bit weird, like me (he's a doctor in New York and I see him perhaps every ten years). Lennie was a violin player, a scholarly young man, very intellectual—you know, the kind of guy that others tease because they're different. One day, when we were fourth-year medical students, Lennie called me up and said that he'd met a girl that I ought to know. I was about 185 pounds and 6 feet tall then and was beginning to feel sure of myself. I had dated girls, but had never dated someone intelligent until he introduced me to Lenore Schwartz. She was a college student majoring in anthropology at Northwestern, an only child of a middle-class family. They owned an automobile and had a nice apartment, and she could afford to go to Northwestern University, which was way beyond my reach.

"Lenore used to talk about poetry and Shakespeare, pretty heavy stuff for a young medical student. I couldn't wait to see her and do all the things that she wanted to do. She was a very affectionate, feminine, scholarly lady, and we were totally in love.

"When I became an intern, she was a graduate student and did her thesis on psychological testing in backward countries. She was a heavyweight intellectual. As an intern, I used to work thirty-six hours on and twelve hours off, and it was tough for us to get together. We felt we had to get married in order to see each other. Because she was so close to her parents, Lenore thought that we should go and ask them for her hand. They were good people; I really loved Lenore's parents, and they had practically adopted me. We sat down and Lenore said, 'Mom and Dad, Emil and I are going to get married.' They said, 'Oh, that's wonderful,' and we had a drink. But then they said, 'Lenore, you're in your third year of graduate school in Evanston, and, Emil, you're in the Cook County Hospital. You can't live in the Medical Center, what are you going to do about school?' After a couple of hours of discussion it was clear that they were opposed to our marriage. That evening I slept at their house, as I sometimes did if I stayed late, and I remember that after everyone retired, Lenore got up in the middle of the night and came to my room and we had a very sad conversation. She said we couldn't elope because she loved her parents. We decided that we'd stay the way we were and not get married.

"What happened to us during the year is what happens often during an internship year; as I said, interns work thirty-six hours on and twelve hours off and the twelve hours that we were off we'd try to screw the nurses who worked on the ward or in the operating room, get drunk, and smoke cigarettes, and then do the thirty-six hours again. I'd see Lenore once in two or three months and the first thing you know I'm hitting it off pretty damn well with one of the student nurses and the relationship with Lenore became strained. At the same time Lenore was being pulled to Northwestern activities and parties. She accused me of dating other girls and not seeing enough of her. The next thing I knew we had broken up. We decided not to get married and to go our separate ways.

"She started dating another guy, but there wasn't a lot to that relationship from her point of view. Then, six months after we decided that we weren't going to get married, Lenore found out that she had acute leukemia. Her parents were very bitter about the whole thing. When I called her mother and father and asked to visit Lenore, they told me that she was through with me. Everyone dumped their guilt on me and in effect said, 'You were cruel to Lenore, and that's how she got leukemia.' You know how families are."

Lenore was one of the first patients with leukemia to receive steroids, and she did go into remission for a time. During the period of the remission, J arranged to meet her. They had coffee together, and Lenore told J that her parents would be very unhappy if they knew that she was seeing him at all.

"It was bitter and painful, really horrible for me and I think for her, too. She died without ever loving that other guy. She really loved me and I loved her. We had wanted to get married in the worst way, but events conspired so that, when she died, I wasn't able to be at her side. Her parents wouldn't allow me to see her and wouldn't allow me to come and grieve, and they continued to be very bitter toward me. It was very, very painful for me and very, very ugly. But I had forgotten all about that until now. It never occurred to me that Lenore Schwartz may have played a role in my going into leukemia research. And yet, when I went to Boston and Joe Ross had leukemia patients that he didn't want to take care of because he thought it was more important to work on anemia, I took care of them. Then when I went to NIH and Zubrod asked me if I wanted to work on leukemia, I said, 'Of course.'

"There's a curious and ironic postscript to the story. Lenore's family memorialized her by founding the research publication *Leukemia Abstracts*: they did this with their own money and money that they raised from the community. I have every issue that was ever published for seventeen years before the funding ran out. It provided leukemia researchers with information about research in leukemia from the international medical literature. On the front page was a lithograph that she had done—she was both an artist and an anthropologist. When you turned over the front page, there was a photograph of her and a little write-up about her life and her tragic death in the middle of a brilliant career. And that hit my desk every month for fifteen years when I was at the NIH. Wow!"

All of this happened before J ever conducted his first experiment with leukemia. If he had any illusions about making a rapid or spectacular breakthrough, he was soon disappointed. Rather, Dr. Zubrod suggested to him that he begin by working with leukemia patients and develop a set of criteria for defining the nature of a clinical response. It wasn't sufficient to say that the patient was better; that was like describing Cyrano as having a big nose. Rather, you needed to be able to evaluate the condition by objective measurements so that someone in another institution could understand your criteria and reproduce your results. Consequently, every bit of research that J Freireich and Tom Frei did with patients was carefully measured and recorded—a direct result of Zubrod's influence.

Expressing data in quantitative and statistical terms was not glamorous work, but it became a way of life. J, Tom, and their colleagues developed the first randomized clinical trials in this country—for any treatment, for any disease—a very important advance in therapeutic research. By this technique the researcher could compare two treatments that, as far as anyone knew, might be equally good, but one was the best standard treatment and the other was new. The patient who agreed to participate in the study would be assigned to receive either of the two forms of treatment according to chance alone. The patient would be treated according to a predefined protocol. At the end of the study, the numerical results would be analyzed by statisticians who did not know which of the treatments the patient received. They would only know that the patient received either treatment "A" or treatment "B." This is now accepted as the critical way of testing any new therapeutic strategy in all fields of medical research.

The team's very first clinical trial compared leukemic children treated with 6-azauracil with those who received no specific chemotherapy. This was done only with children who had failed to respond to the other drugs available at that time. In a few patients the blood counts did improve, but the patients quickly relapsed. When J and his colleagues wrote up their results, the reviewer for the journal criticized the ethics of doing placebo trials on such patients. By contrast, today if you wrote a paper claiming the effectiveness of a new drug and you *failed* to have a randomized placebo control, you'd be criticized on ethical grounds. Fashions change drastically, even in science. Taking care of the human problem never does.

That 6-azauracil trial stands out vividly in my own memory because I took care of some of those children at NCI in 1956. This drug, like others tested in humans, had shown anticancer effects in animals. But in humans the drug had a very peculiar side effect; some patients slept for days and even went into coma while they were taking the drug and for some days after stopping. Even patients who didn't go into deep sleep or coma had abnormal brain waves: although they were walking around the ward, their brain waves were the same as if they had been asleep. I've never seen anything like it before or since. It was probably fair to conclude from that very early study that not only was 6-azauracil an inactive compound against human leukemia, but the patients on the placebo did better than those on the drug. Yet this was clear only because J and his colleagues had insisted on including a placebo group of patients.

"It proves the obvious—that not everything you have a good reason to try in patients is successful. But the next study we did was considerably more successful: we studied whether newly treated patients, that is, those that hadn't previously been treated with chemotherapy, would have their remissions prolonged if we treated them even while they *were* in remission. The strategy was to treat all of the patients with a steroid called prednisone to get as many into remission as possible. We knew that this remission would have only a short duration, but then we could take patients who were freshly in remission and randomly assign them to receive a chemotherapeutic drug. In this case either they were given 6-MP or they received no further treatment until they relapsed. Then we could ask whether the patients stayed in remission longer if they were treated continuously with 6-MP. The answer could not be predicted in advance of doing the study. Doctors Skipper and Schabel had worked out such a model in animals, but I was really the first to propose that you could 'cure' cancer only by treating patients while they were in remission.

"Now we come to the good part of the story. When we gave the 6-MP to patients who had achieved a remission after treatment with prednisone, the remission would last about thirty weeks. Thus half of the children were living longer than the longest surviving patients had lived before without being treated with some other therapy. It seemed that the group of patients benefited from being treated with 6-MP while they were in remission—even patients who might not have responded had the single drug [6-MP] been given to them without previous prednisone.

''This is the kind of project that Tom Frei and I worked out. I so admire Tom because he's such an intellectual and many of these ideas were his. Although Tom and I had originally come in at the same level of appointment about the same time, Tom became my boss—but he was never bossy. He always helped me but never told me what to do, and I had total confidence in him. We discussed everything for hours. Everybody trusted Tom even if they didn't trust me because I tended to be flamboyant. When I would come up with some outrageous idea, Zubrod would tell me that I was crazy. But Frei would say, 'Well, you know how he is. It *is* an outrageous idea, but why don't we try it?'

"Zubrod was really the Eisenhower of the National Cancer Institute. He kept getting promoted, and he created the freedom for us to do our work and expand our horizons. However, he believed that, if you do everything, you will also know everything. I didn't believe that. Consequently I was often in the doghouse with Zubrod. Nevertheless, he handled other administrative hurdles that we might not have surmounted otherwise. For example, we had a number of single drugs that could work for a time in patients with leukemia, but eventually the patients relapsed and died. The beginning of the use of combinations of drugs really depended on a class of drugs called the vinca alkaloids, a family of compounds that are derived from the very common periwinkle plant. Eli Lilly, the pharmaceutical company known for its work with other natural products such as insulin, was the center of drug development of these compounds. One of their young Ph.D.s, Irv Johnson, had found that a crude vinca alkaloid mixture was no use against the mouse leukemia model L_{1210}. However, it did cure one type of lymphoma in mice, and Johnson told the Lilly board that he thought they had an exciting drug.

"The Lilly scientists proceeded to purify the mixture, and they ended up with two active anticancer drugs, vinblastine and vincristine. In trials in Indianapolis, they found that vincristine had some antitumor effects in patients with lymphoma. The strange thing about vincristine was that it had some peculiar toxicity against the nervous system, though no toxicity on normal blood cells. That was very unusual because chemotherapeutic drugs characteristically inhibit blood cell production. The Lilly investigators showed us their data on improvement in three cases of Hodgkin's disease. At that time Dr. Zubrod didn't want to do any clinical trials in patients with acute leukemia unless the drug had been effective in treating mice with leukemia, which this drug hadn't. However, I felt that, since we had numerous children who had relapsed following the best chemotherapy available, we should try vincristine. Zubrod said that it was OK if we wanted to do it, but that he was opposed to the idea. This was a trait I admired in him; he would disagree with you, yet not impose his views on you. So he let me proceed, and in the first ten or eleven patients who had failed to respond to other drugs we had several who had complete remissions. That was impressive!"

Frei and Freireich's paper on their observations that vincristine was active against childhood leukemia, along with Zubrod and Frei's eleventh-hour trip to Indianapolis (see Chapter 7), came just in the nick of time to revive Eli Lilly's faltering drug development program. Ultimately it became a very profitable drug for the company. The important point about vincristine was that it had both antileukemia activity *and* a toxicity that differed from the other drugs used. It was thus possible to use full doses of the other drugs while adding vincristine, because vincristine's toxicity would not add to the toxic side effects of the other drugs. Instead, it would manifest its toxicity in some other area of the body. That was really the beginning of *combination chemotherapy*. The key was that the researchers were able to give each of the drugs in full doses.

"We had carefully worked out everything on paper. Tom Frei probably deserves most of the credit for this. Most of the things that I did between 1955 and 1972 were done jointly with Tom Frei. He's the brains, but we were truly synergistic. After we had worked out this protocol, Zubrod at first thought it would be too toxic, but again he allowed us to proceed and in that sense he was the real hero."

Before proceeding with the chemotherapy part of J's story, we need to pause and consider a series of other discoveries that had to occur before the chemotherapy could ever be curative. Prior to the creation of the leukemia ward at the National Cancer Institute, medical scientists thought that they understood the disease of acute leukemia. However, Gordon Zubrod hoped that studying the subtle variations in the expression of the disease would provide important clues on how to devise effective strategies for curing it. He had no way of knowing whether this approach would be successful, of course. But by focusing so much talent in his group on the leukemia patients, many new discoveries were made about the nature of the disease even while new methods of drug treatment were being tested.

The decision by Zubrod to study the clinical features of leukemia turned out later to have a crucial influence on its treatment. A couple of examples from the late 1950s are illustrative. Many children with leukemia died very suddenly when the disease relapsed. The first breakthrough discovery, made around 1958 by J, Tom, and a number of very able young clinical associates, was that this type of sudden death could be predicted when the child had a severe relapse and a rapidly rising leukemic cell count, say, in excess of 300,000 per cubic millimeter of blood (normal is 5,000 to 10,000 white cells). Death came, as Freireich and others recognized, when blood vessels plugged up with leukemic cells hemorrhaged into the brain. But the group also demonstrated that the fatal hemorrhage could be averted by rapidly lowering the cell count.

Next they learned that, contrary to the advice of neurologists who felt it was too dangerous, it was vital to do a spinal fluid puncture in children with leukemia who had altered consciousness in order to diagnose the problem correctly, such as whether it was a type of meningitis, or hemorrhage. By so doing, the proper treatment could be started. Also, only in this way could we appreciate the frequency of serious involvement of leukemia in the lining (meninges) of brain and spinal cord, problems that actually became more frequent as patients began to live longer. These very important observations that saved many lives around the world were finally published in 1960 in *Neurology* after having been rejected by three journals.

Freireich and others subsequently worked out the effectiveness of putting folate antagonists directly into the spinal fluid to control meningeal leukemia: this in turn set the stage for the prophylactic administration of drugs into the spinal fluid to prevent the occurrence of leukemia in the brain as opposed to treating it once it had occurred. This was to become a key element in the cure of childhood leukemia.

The unfolding of the story about the cause of yet another crucial clinical problem, that of generalized bleeding in patients with leukemia, was so interesting, tense, and controversial that we should hear directly from J himself, the central figure in this scientific drama.

"When I arrived for my first day of work at the NCI, Tom Frei said, 'Here are three patients with leukemia who are left over from Jim Holland. Nobody knows what to do with them, so why don't you take them over?' So I said OK. When everybody realized that I liked caring for these kids, we began to get some referrals and I went out and gave some medical lectures and built up a proper leukemia service in a couple of months. Dr. Zubrod used to come on rounds regularly, and one day he said, 'You know, Freireich, every patient on your ward has blood splattered all over the linens—I think this bleeding is very important.' Indeed it was very evident to everybody that in the mid-1950s some 90 percent of the patients with childhood leukemia died of hemorrhage. And then Zubrod said, 'You're a hematologist, why don't you go to work on this hemorrhage problem?'

"The first thing I did was what anyone would do: read all the literature. But knowledge about hemorrhage and leukemia was still fairly limited. In 1953 Dr. George Brecher and Dr. Eugene Cronkite at NCI had invented the phase microscope method of counting platelets, which finally let us count platelets accurately. Their experiments in dogs had shown unequivocally that, when you transfused blood, the platelets would circulate for a time, and that the platelets were necessary in controlling hemorrhage. Then Isaac Djerassi, Edmond Klein, and their colleagues in Boston had found that extracts of frozen platelets (not whole platelets) stopped hemorrhage in children. Well, there was a large and complicated literature on platelet extracts and their peculiar effects on blood clotting in the test tube and in the whole body, but still no one had solved the problem, so Freireich had to solve it.

"Again I did what any young person would do. I started from square one and collected blood samples from all the children who were bleeding, took the blood to my laboratory, and measured everything I could that might conceivably be relevant. I measured all of the classical tests of bleeding and platelet function, and I found that everything that was wrong with the children's blood when the children were bleeding could be corrected by adding concentrates of platelets, whether the platelets were alive or dead. All I needed was platelet stuff. The question was, 'I want to get the active material out of platelets, how do I do it?' Ed Korn at the Heart Institute taught me how to use the ultracentrifuge to separate platelets and to obtain a fraction, the so-called platelet factor 3. When I found that it completely corrected the bleeding tendency in the test tube, I wanted to give it to children. We went through all the shenanigans of 'You can't do it, you've got to give it to animals and do toxicity studies first in animals, you've got to kill the mice and see what it does to the mice.' But I said that was a total waste of time, it's a human product, I was going to give it to humans. It seemed totally safe, and I'd done all of the test-tube kinds of tests and if I kept on doing all the things they told me to do it would take five years and I'd be dead!

"As usual, Tom Frei said, 'Freireich's crazy, but Zubrod won't interfere, why don't you go ahead and give it to one patient?' So I did. I made my platelet extract from volunteer donors and injected the platelet factor 3 into a bleeding patient, and the bleeding stopped immediately. But the *duration* of the effect was only about five minutes. It was obvious from studying the blood what had happened. The platelet factor 3 is quickly cleared out of the blood system within minutes, even in the sickest child. As long as I'm shooting the stuff into the patient, the bleeding stops, but as soon as I stop injecting it, it gets cleared out of the bloodstream and the effect is gone. So the answer was to give it continuously—but I couldn't make that much platelet extract.

"Whatever the solution to the problem of hemorrhage in children, this obviously wasn't it. So I argued that, what I can do with extracts of platelets, I can do better with whole platelets, so I'll transfuse whole platelets. But Dr. Brecher, chief of the Laboratory Service and who had done that early platelet research, told me that platelets wouldn't work: if you give platelets more than once they cause sensitization, and that sensitization reaction is so important that never would you give people platelets because in the end it would be ineffective. So I said, 'Goddamn it! I do it in a test tube and I do it every time: it's got to work in people.'

"I went back to Tom and he said, 'You can't do it, you've got to give it to animals first; besides, Brecher won't allow it. Dr. Schmidt runs the blood bank, and it's illegal, and the director of the Cancer Institute, Dr. Mider, won't allow it,' and so on.

"We knew they wouldn't allow it under any circumstances even if I took a blood donor and prepared the platelets myself. It was illegal! So we worked out this scheme.

"Tom and I decided to do a prospective randomized study in which we would give whole blood to children with leukemia who were bleeding; half of them would get the ordinary whole blood that had been refrigerated and kept in the blood bank, while the other half would receive fresh blood from donors. The refrigeration clumps and destroys the platelets, but freshly drawn, unrefrigerated blood would keep the platelets in a live form and they should then be effective. We would code the transfusions so that the doctors giving the blood and those measuring whether or not the patient stopped bleeding and also the persons who were doing the platelet count would not know whether the patients got fresh blood or stored bank blood. That was our plan to try to prove the effectiveness of platelets.

"Meanwhile, I kept after Dr. Schmidt to get me straight platelets, and the director of the Cancer Institute called me up and said, 'If you don't stop harassing Dr. Schmidt, I'm going to fire you.' I wanted to give platelets to children who were bleeding, and Brecher knew that was wrong, Schmidt knew that was wrong, and there were a hundred articles in the literature that said it wouldn't work—and yet I had the audacity to insist.

"The issue came to a head at a grand rounds at the Clinical Center building. I presented my data on the clotting time and the bleeding time on so many patients and the test-tube evaluation results. I said I wanted to give the patients platelets. Brecher got up, reviewed what he and Cronkite had found, and said it would be inappropriate to give platelets. Then Schmidt got up and gave more data that indicated that giving platelets was a bad idea. At the end of the meeting, Dr. Schmidt declared that no one in the Clinical Center would ever get fresh blood because it was known to be potentially harmful and it wouldn't work. Now Gordon Zubrod believed Brecher and Schmidt, and he had told me to my face that he thought I was wrong. But he was amazing—we're not talking about a man who was simply expressing his views, he was a man operating on principle. He went to the microphone and said, 'Dr. Brecher, I've listened to this grand rounds, and I want to say one thing in public. I am clinical director, and the leukemia patients are my responsibility, and Dr. Freireich reports to me. If any of my doctors order fresh platelets, you'll deliver them as long as it's my responsibility to see to it that it's provided.' And he sat down and the place went nuts! And I told Tom Frei that Zubrod was a giant. So the double-blind study was proposed as a compromise. Brecher and Schmidt agreed, probably because they were convinced it wouldn't work; we agreed because we thought it would.

"It was the first randomized controlled study of this subject in which half the bleeding patients would receive fresh blood and half stored bank blood. And no one would break the code as to which was which until we agreed to do it in public. [The 'code' is what makes it a blind experiment. Breaking the code reveals the results *and* the treatment, or nontreatment, that produced the results.] There we all were in the room—Schmidt, Brecher, Frei, Freireich, and the statistician Marvin Schneiderman—when it came time to break open the code. Schmidt, the director of the blood bank, knew which product had been given to the patient. Brecher had done the platelet counts, but he didn't know what the patient had received. Freireich had done the clinical evaluation, but he didn't know what the patient had gotten, and so on. And furthermore Schmidt didn't know what the results of the transfusions had been, that is, whether the bleeding had stopped in the transfused patients, although he had obtained the blood from the donors. It was all carefully blinded and recorded objectively.

"The code was revealed like this: Someone would say, 'Dr. Freireich, patient number so and so, please report the bleeding effect after we gave transfusion number 1.' And I would report the change in the status of the patient, and whether the bleeding had stopped completely or partially or not at all, and at what time. We put all the clinical data on the blackboard. Step two, 'Dr. Schmidt, please reveal the source of the blood.' Guess what? 100 percent of those patients whose bleeding stopped were patients who had received fresh blood, including its active platelets. By the time we had gone through fifteen patients, the difference was already statistically significant. There was no likelihood of confusion. Oh my God, can you believe it?

"So what do you think they did next?

"Well, they said I cheated! Dr. Brecher went to Dr. Zubrod and said, 'We know how this study was done. Family members were called to the blood bank to give fresh blood, and later Dr. Freireich interviewed them and thereby found out that they had been donors of the fresh blood. He falsified the clinical data and that's why the correlations were good.' And so Dr. Brecher refused to put his name on the research manuscript that described the work. Now Tom Frei didn't know what to do and Gordon Zubrod didn't know what to do. How did they know that I didn't cheat? This was my first big research project, I'm a young crazy guy, and the others are older experts who were sure they were right. Eventually there was a public confrontation, and I denied any wrongdoing. I pointed out that my fellows had been instructed not to interview the families, and I certainly did not, and they just had to take that as my word. Tom Frei defended me, and Zubrod said that he'd made rounds with me a hundred times and knew me to be an honest person: if I said I didn't cheat, then he knew I didn't cheat.

"A neutral judge, another scientist in the Medicine Branch of NCI, held a kind of inquisition. The big decision to be made was whether the material should be submitted to a journal: it might humiliate the institution to publish controversial data that had been accused of being falsified. The meeting ended with Tom Frei saying that he'd put his name on the paper because he believed the response; he'd been present during the breaking of the blinded study and he'd been present with me over the year that this study was conducted and so his name would go on the paper. Furthermore, he proposed that anyone who didn't believe the data should take his name off the paper, which then would be handled through the usual academic process. If you look at that paper, you'll see who had the courage to put his name on it. Marvin Schneiderman's name is on it, Tom Frei's name is on it, and in the end, Paul Schmidt's too. Brecher is the one who didn't put his name on it, and he and I didn't talk for about ten years after that."

"The *New England Journal of Medicine* accepted the paper. When it was published in 1959, it created havoc! But while all this process of review and publication was going on, there was a delay of four or five months, and in the meantime I had to take the next step. I had done platelet counts on all those children, so I correlated the platelet counts themselves with the presence or absence of hemorrhage. The paper that an NCI fellow, Dr. Gaydos, a statistician, Marvin Schneiderman, and I published on it is considered a citation classic in the field, together with the first paper on the platelets. We were able to show that the platelet count correlated directly with the clinical events, objectively and quantitatively. Patients didn't bleed unless and until their platelet count dropped to very low levels—then they were likely to have bleeding episodes. Gaydos went through all the records of the doctors, nurses, social workers, and whatever else was available that described bleeding, and he correlated them with the platelet count.

"We were technically able to measure smaller increases in platelet counts than had ever been done before, down to 5,000 platelets per microliter. No one had come close to doing that before. Can you imagine my audacity when I gave a paper at the annual meetings in Atlantic City and the internationally renowned hematologist Bill Dameshek got up and said, 'I can't tell the difference between 5,000 or 20,000 platelets, so how can you make these claims?' "

I was in the audience at that tense moment. The huge "Steel Pier" auditorium was packed with doctors, many standing up in the back. J's rejoinder to Dr. Dameshek was stunning: "I agree that *you* can't tell the difference, but I can, because we don't use the Dameshek method [of counting platelets]; we use the phase contrast method." Dameshek's very indirect method for counting these tiny platelets was only accurate to $\pm 50,000$ platelets per microliter. Here was young Dr. Freireich, asserting that a difference of a mere 5,000 to 20,000 in the platelet count was the difference between bleeding and not bleeding spontaneously. That was a radical claim. It was the only time I've ever seen the loquacious Dr. Dameshek speechless.

"It wasn't meant to be impertinent. It was meant to be responsive to the question. You see, George Brecher had shown earlier that, by measuring the platelets with the phase microscope under heated (body temperature) conditions, you could easily see the difference between a platelet count of 1,000 and that of 6,000. I did the platelet counts in my own lab with my own eyes and knew that I could tell the difference.

"Anyway, now I was really excited. If as few as 5,000 platelets per cubic millimeter of blood was enough to stop the bleeding, good grief, what would happen if we gave patients two units of blood and that many more platelets?"

In the meantime, Paul Schmidt left the NIH and the blood bank was turned over to Dr. Alan Kliman. Immediately, J approached him. "The wicked witch of the east is dead, and now you're in charge of the blood bank, aren't you?"

"Yes, sir," Al said.

"Well, listen, Al," J responded, "I have this idea about transfusing platelets. We gave bleeding leukemic children one unit of fresh blood, and now I'm wondering what would happen if, instead, we gave them two units of platelets. You understand what I want to do is to just give them units of platelets and throw away the red cells."

Because a 30-kilogram (66-pound) child has only four units of blood altogether, a transfusion of just one unit of fresh whole blood would displace a substantial part of the child's total blood volume. *Two* units of whole blood would be overwhelming. But just the platelets from two units would not change the volume significantly.

What was needed was to fractionate the blood into its component parts, and particularly to isolate the living platelets for transfusion into the child. Dr. Kliman had learned a technique of fractionation that made it possible to take the red blood cells out of the transfusion, or put them back, simply by using a special plastic blood bag. He could put a unit of fresh blood into the centrifuge, choose the right speed, and spin out the platelets that remained in the plasma and separate them from the denser red blood cells.

"Alan worked this out and we talked about it over barbecued hamburgers in his backyard. We developed a sterile closed system whereby we connected two [Fenwal] plastic bloodbags with a little 'Y' type connector that you could buy from a plastics manufacturer. You could push the plasma out of one sterile bag into another and then separate the bags. Then you could go and give the red blood cells back to the donor and keep the platelets to give to the patient. Everybody thought we were nuts, so we just went about our business. Then I said, 'Look, Kliman, why should we give just one or two units of platelets? Why don't we give the kids enough platelets to get their platelet counts back to normal and see if they get sensitized to them, as the experts predicted?' "

Naturally, the first question that had to be asked about this ingenious procedure was how many units of platelets a normal donor could give without being hurt in any way. Theoretically, there should be no harm from removing platelets repeatedly from the same individual because they are built back up again rather quickly.

One blood volume in a normal adult is approximately five liters of blood—red blood cells make up some 45 percent and plasma about 55 percent. The fraction that includes white blood cells (like granulocytes) and platelets accounts for less than 1 percent of the volume. If one full blood volume of red blood cells were to be removed, there would be none left for the donor: however, since the granulocytes within the blood compartment are in equilibrium with other granulocytes in the tissues (bone marrow, along blood vessels), removal of one full volume of granulocytes only results in a partial and temporary fall in the granulocyte count. Similarly, the procedure lowered platelet counts only temporarily. The rest of the blood volume was transferred back to the donor. Hence granulocytes, and also platelets, could be continuously removed (up to a point) from the blood without any danger whatever to the donor.

J, his NCI fellow Bob Levin (who, sadly, later died in a plane crash), and Kliman soon found that they could remove four units of platelets a week indefinitely from a normal person without causing any ill effects. Then Dr. Levin set out to make a platelet concentrate that combined the platelets from the equivalent of four conventional units of whole blood (or two liters), which could now be obtained from a single healthy donor.

Family members and friends, of course, were only too happy to be donors for these leukemic children. Being able to get so many units of platelets from a single individual was a great advantage. A single donor could provide roughly 400 billion platelets, which, it turned out, would raise the platelet count of an average child by about 100,000. Freireich, Kliman, and Levin planned a prospective randomized study that would compare one versus two versus four versus five units of platelets.

"But on further reflection I said, 'Let's cut the crap and just eliminate hemorrhage.' And Kliman said, 'I'm like you, let's just eliminate the hemorrhage.' And he told me that, if I could get the donors, he'd give me the platelets whenever I needed them. Whenever a patient anywhere on the whole Leukemia Service began to hemorrhage, we measured the platelet count. If it was low, we transfused platelets. Gordon Zubrod came on rounds one day and he said, 'You know, Freireich, I remember the first days we made rounds here and all the kids had blood on their pillows. Now I don't see any blood on any pillows.' That made me feel good. I had made a rule on the Leukemia Service that, if I ever spotted a patient bleeding, the fellow responsible would get axed. There was not a single patient who didn't respond to the platelets.

"We did have patients who became sensitized to platelets, the problem that Brecher had predicted would be our Achilles heel. We had to develop special techniques to give them even more platelets, but in all cases we overcame the bleeding. And we proved it in one shot—bingo! Just like that! I wrote a paper and sent it to the *Journal of Clinical Investigation* (*JCI*). I'll never forget it because the paper was rejected. My goal in life was to become an academic. To get that kind of job, I had to publish in the *JCI*, and here my important paper was rejected.

"A friend on the editorial board of the *Journal* looked into it and told me the paper was simply too practical and clinical for the *JCI*. I said to him, 'Bill, what is going on here? This is the most important clinical research that I will ever do. This is exciting. It flies in the face of all the conventional wisdom of twenty years of platelet research. How can the *JCI* turn it down?' He just repeated that it was too practical.

"I finally sent it to the *Annals of Internal Medicine* in 1963 and they published it, even though some referees gave it horrible reviews. We were criticized for not having done a prospective randomized control study. What I had done instead was to compare each patient's count before and after the platelet transfusion, and I could account for all of the increases entirely by the transfusion of the platelets. I'd done thousands of them, so I knew the story exactly. All I had to do was to plot the results. There's a famous figure in that paper which has since been quoted quite extensively, but at that time it was still very controversial—though to me it was conclusive. It was the first time we had used so-called historical controls, that is, to compare the same patient before and after treatment, and the difference was so obvious. Yet everyone wanted me to do a randomized trial in which half of the patients got platelets, but I didn't do that. That's the end of the story except for the fact that Scott Murphy and other scientists elsewhere did a very good job of finding better ways of preserving the fragile platelets and of keeping them viable for transfusion.

"But ours was the start of platelet research because, from then on, you could use platelets. And they worked."

Freireich did not stop there in his quest to keep leukemia patients alive long enough to respond to chemotherapy. Now that he had figured out how to stop the fatal hemorrhaging, the next task was preventing deadly infections.

"Alan Kliman and I were barbecuing in his backyard just as we had when we devised the bags for transfusion, and he said, 'You know,

Freireich, now that you've controlled hemorrhage, 90 percent of the children who die are dying of infection. Why don't you do something about that?' So with the help of one of our junior people, Dr. Gerry Bodey, we did a clinical study of fever and documented that fever and infection, as a cause of death in leukemic children, was closely related to the number of these white cells called granulocytes in the blood. (That study was another citation classic.) Of course, we knew that a shortage of normal infection-fighting granulocytes was the problem for these leukemic children. What they needed was more of the normal white cells. So Al said, 'You know, we did this thing with giving platelets to patients who were deficient in them. Why don't we do the same thing with granulocytes?' "

The idea was sound, but making it work was not so easy. Unlike platelets or red blood cells that circulate freely through the blood, granulocytes tend to congregate along the walls of the blood vessels. Any rise in the granulocyte count obtained after transfusing granulocytes is far less than one might predict based on the number of cells actually transfused. Furthermore, normal people have relatively few granulocytes in their blood, so taking out three, four, six, or eight units of blood or their equivalent in granulocytes would not make much of a difference in a leukemic patient who was devoid of these cells. Freireich and Kliman pondered the problem.

"Could we continuously remove white blood cells from donors? That probably wouldn't work. But then a stroke of genius hit us, and I'm not sure if it was Alan's idea or mine. We knew that patients with chronic granulocytic leukemia have granulocyte counts a hundred times greater than normal and that their granulocytes function pretty well in killing bacteria. One unit of blood from a patient with this kind of leukemia would have 10^{11} granulocytes—more than you'd get from the entire blood volume of a normal person. What if we took two units of white cells from patients with chronic granulocytic leukemia and then gave them to the kids who were low on white blood cells?

"Guess what happened? Zubrod said, 'It's impossible, you have to do it in dogs or in cows first.' Tom Frei sat with me for two days and said, 'J, you cannot do that. You can't give chronic leukemia cells to a child; you'll either give them a different kind of leukemia or transfer a virus. It's insane, you cannot do this! You've got to do it in cows.' And I said, 'Tom, cows don't accept human white cells, they are promptly rejected by the immune system.' Dr. Frank Gardner had done dog studies with granulocytes for years; he'd worked out how to separate them, preserve them, and transfuse them. He had done the first experiments transfusing them into humans and the result was zero. And I said, 'Look, it ain't gonna work in animals. You've got to work on patients because they have a totally different physiology. If I work on humans, I've got to give it to humans.'

"Finally, after all the usual kind of fighting and hemming and hawing and talk about toxicity and danger, they said, 'All right, we'll allow you to give 10cc of granulocytic leukemic blood to the first patient. So we gave this *tiny* amount without incident, and more the next time, and we counted the cells: eventually we got up to the point of giving them two bags, 10^{11} cells of granulocytes from a patient with chronic leukemia—which is what I wanted to do in the first place. It turned out that to get a normal granulocyte count, you had to give them 10^{11} granulocytes. We worked out all the details.

"When we got to the 10^{11} dose Dr. Ed Morse, my fellow at the time, and I started to treat patients. Lo and behold, all of the children who had fever and bloodstream infection were promptly cured of their infection! By giving the chronic granulocytic leukemia cells to children with acute lymphocytic leukemia, we raised their granulocyte counts from nearly zero up to 2,500 per microliter, which is normal. So we published a very famous figure in which we showed response to infection as a function of the dose (number) of the transfused cells. It was a beautiful dose-response effect, and it didn't need any controls. When we were able to achieve a granulocyte count of 2,500, ten out of eleven infected children so treated were cured; with a count of 1,500, seven were cured; and when the count got below 500 granulocytes, only one of eleven children responded. It was very clean data."

[Tom Frei recalls the events rather differently. They had just given a platelet transfusion to a leukemic child from a donor who had polycythemia vera. In the next bed was a patient with chronic leukemia and a very high (300,000 cells per cubic microliter) number of granulocytes that should help cure infection. "It was a quick intellectual leap by analogy which J and I discussed, and the first white cell transfusion was given within two or three days of that observation and discussion."]

Freireich and his colleagues recognized that there was much more work to do on the problem, because there were not many potential white blood cell donors among patients who had chronic granulocyte leukemia, and that certainly wasn't going to solve the problem of low granulocyte count in patients with childhood leukemia. There weren't enough chronic leukemia patients with high counts to act as donors, and making the donations might not have been good treatment for them anyway: the answer simply wasn't known. The next challenge was to get sufficient numbers of granulocytes from perfectly normal donors, but how would one go about doing that?

"That's when I met George Judson, an engineer from IBM. George had a son who had chronic granulocytic leukemia at the time, and George was referred to me by one of my colleagues, Jerry Block, who had told him that Freireich was crazy and he wanted to do this crazy thing. Judson said that he was committed to his son's survival and would do anything he could for research, even if it might be too late to help his son.

"IBM gave him a sabbatical year because they thought he was going to crack up with his son being treated for leukemia. He came to my office and said, 'What is this idea of yours all about?' I had this problem, I told him. I wanted to give 10^{11} normal granulocytes to children who were infected because they lacked granulocytes. It would take the equivalent of two full blood volumes from a normal donor to get that many granulocytes. I wanted to build a new type of centrifuge that would process these blood volumes in a reasonable period of time, harvest off all of the granulocytes, and give all of the other cells and plasma back to the donor. He said, "OK, I'll go to work on it," and he did. IBM paid his salary and he worked at the NIH as a visiting scientist in my laboratory. At the end of his year, we had a prototype machine, but it was a catastrophe, because it wouldn't work. Nonetheless, we thought we knew exactly how to clear up the technical problems and resolve the design flaws. We persuaded NCI to write a contract with IBM that gave us access to all of the company's resources to solve those difficult technical problems.

"It took more than a year, perhaps a year and a half to crack the problem. I personally conducted the first clinical trial with the new instrument, and it was a total failure. So I called Judson into my office and said, 'George, guess what, the machine doesn't work.' The pumps were supposed to deliver blood on a continuous basis, but the face seals on the pumps were leaking. The red cells were going into the white cell area where they didn't belong, and I couldn't get the proper separation of blood components. We had spent $500,000 on the machine, and we had a total failure.

I told Judson that 'I wasn't going to go f—— around on a patient with a machine that could not consistently pump the blood and until we could test it satisfactorily in the laboratory with blood from the blood bank. Go and do it in the goddamn laboratory.'

"I suspended the clinical trials, and unfortunately Judson was humiliated. IBM had a company policy that any engineer who failed to deliver on a contract would be fired immediately. Judson panicked, went to Zubrod, and said, 'Freireich is unreasonable, and he has to be fired.' Tom Frei called me into his office and told me, 'Freireich, I know it's wrong, but Zubrod has decided that you've got to leave this project. We're going to make Dr. Seymour Perry the project officer, and the IBM people will work with him.' So everybody put on a good face so that it looked as if IBM hadn't failed and gave IBM another $100,000 for another year, and Dr. Perry worked with them. But they never tried it on a patient and the project never went anywhere.

"I pleaded with Tom that it was all my concept, my idea, my thought, my energy, and without me nothing would happen. He said he knew that, but it had to be done, otherwise the whole thing would have blown up. So I said, 'Fine, if you have to do it, do it.' I'm sure the politics of it were the same reason he left NCI in 1965 for M. D. Anderson Hospital in Houston. I moved there myself a few months later.

"The NCI people worked on the cell separator for two or three years after that, but made no progress. Then one day, George Judson appeared in my office in Houston and he said, 'Guess what? The contract has just ended at NCI and there's nothing going on.' And I said, 'Well, what are you talking to me for?' And he said, 'We think we've solved the problem you told us to solve.' I was working at a new hospital and had new problems to think about. Still, when Judson appeared, I admit I was interested. They had learned to put a salt solution at the interface between the little channels on the seal; if the seals came apart, the salt solution would keep the fractions of blood separated. It really worked! They had also redesigned the pump. George said, 'Nothing will happen at IBM, because Perry doesn't care about the project. They'll never treat another patient at NCI. I know you care about it, and I've convinced IBM management, rather than abandon the project, to manufacture three prototype machines of the kind that I think will work. We'll place them in other institutions at no cost to the institution. Would you accept one of the machines?' I said of course. Then Judson stepped out of the picture. A businessman came to deliver the machine, and we had a ceremony with the president of the hospital.

"Tommy Daniels, my very good assistant at M. D. Anderson, and I tested the instrument out in the laboratory with blood bank blood and it worked fine. Then it was time to take it to the clinic. First, we processed the blood from a patient with chronic lymphocytic leukemia who had too many leukemic lymphocytes in his blood; we skimmed off the leukemic cells into a separate bag and then gave the patient back all of the normal cells, including red blood cells and platelets. The machine worked like a dream.

"We used a similar procedure for doing granulocyte transfusion, but it never has been as useful as platelet transfusion. Granulocytes do sensitize the recipient, you see, and you get dangerous reactions if you give these white blood cells repeatedly because they collect in the small blood vessels in the lung. And because the cells don't live very long in the circulation, you've got to give at least two doses of granulocytes a day for four days and that's too expensive and too difficult technically. So it never became a useful or practical procedure, but it was very important from a physiological point of view, and we learned a great deal. It does work and we still do it at times."

Most modern hospitals now use blood cell separators for a whole variety of medical applications: research, treatment of patients with leukemia, removing plasma from patients with abnormal serum proteins or certain types of neurological diseases, and so on. In the end, George Judson's work made a major contribution to medical science. Even though it didn't save his son's life, it has contributed to saving the lives of many other people—a source of considerable satisfaction for Judson, Freireich, and the other people who worked on the project.

Of all the projects J undertook at NCI, the one he recalls with the warmest enthusiasm was the combination chemotherapy program. Like so much of J's research, it struck others as far-fetched and crazy to start with. Yet to J it was a logical extension of his earlier chemotherapy work.

From the early 6-MP/vincristine project, it had become clear to J and Tom that it made sense to give drugs in combination rather than in sequence. If the drugs were given in sequence, that is, one after another, those patients who failed to respond to the first drug often died before they had the opportunity to get the second drug. If the drugs were given in combination, however, every patient would have an opportunity to respond to both drugs. For example, when methotrexate was used by itself the remission rate was 30 percent: thus 70 percent of the children failed to respond. Because the disease is so aggressive, 20 percent or more would die before they could be treated by a second drug. J and Tom did the calculations on paper and predicted that, of the 70 percent of children who failed to respond on methotrexate, an extra 15 percent would respond if they were simultaneously treated with 6-MP—and that's exactly what happened. The effect achieved with those two drugs was roughly additive.

If combining methotrexate and 6-MP brought 45 percent of the children into remission, what—J now wanted to know—would happen if *four* antileukemic drugs were given all at once? "I wanted to give full doses of vincristine *and* aminopterin, combined with the 6-MP *and* prednisone." The combination was called VAMP (*V*incristine, *A*methopterin [methotrexate], 6*MP*, *P*rednisone), the first of many acronyms for different chemotherapy combinations.

The study was designed in 1962. Getting it under way, however, required the agreement of all the hospitals in the cooperative groups affiliated with NCI, in order to share resources and to have enough patients to provide statistically reliable results. However, the members of the cooperative group had already made plans to study a different treatment protocol on methotrexate. To stay in the cooperative group, J would have either had to enroll all his NCI patients in a protocol he did not believe in or else persuade the group to try the radically new VAMP study. The situation was complicated by the fact that Tom Frei chaired the cooperative group; even though he supported J's idea, he also had to keep the cooperative group running smoothly.

J decided that his only choice was to pull out of the cooperative group and put all his new NCI patients into his own VAMP study. "It was an impasse that had to be overcome by the passion of one person. It was very difficult for me, because we were proposing something that we knew could bring the whole place down. NCI was a young institute and we'd never really done anything of major experimental proportions before. VAMP was an outrageous idea. It was insane; we could barely do it at NCI, with all our resources. How could any other institution do it? But I felt an urgent need to do it. Why? Because I think that clinical research is a matter of urgency. The people who have the disease now are going to die if you

141

take a year to develop a drug, so why not cure them now? I had patients I cared about. It was the philosophy of Roland P. Woodyatt all over again. Why shouldn't I cure my patients? It had to be done now! I knew these children, I knew their parents, they came to me for help and they wanted me to do something. I felt compelled to do the VAMP study, so that's what I did."

As with Freireich's earlier projects, Gordon Zubrod had serious reservations, both about its experimental method and about its ethics. J always felt that original research on leukemia had to start with observations and experiments in the clinic, with patients: animal model systems were useful afterwards for enlarging on the clinical observations. Zubrod always wanted to work the other way around: start with experiments on animals with leukemia, then try out the results on the ward. This indeed became the standard biomedical approach approved by NCI and the Food and Drug Administration, and J remains highly critical of it.

"I should mention that if you tried to do a clinical study of VAMP today without an experimental basis in animals, even if you were the most powerful clinical scientist in this country, you couldn't do it. The FDA would say you can't give four drugs concurrently to patients until you know what V + A, V + M, and so forth give you. Then you've got to do all of the three possible combinations *and* then you've got to do all of the four combinations *and* with different doses and schedules for each. So to have done VAMP in one giant leap was a real tour de force. But it was hopeless to model this in animals.

"There was no mouse tumor in which all four drugs were effective. Look at the mouse leukemia L_{1210}—the prednisone does nothing to prolong the life of the mice, vincristine does a little bit, 6-MP is slightly active, and methotrexate is the big gun, but even that depends on how you give the drug, whether you treat the mice when they have very early leukemia or if you wait until the leukemia is already advanced. So only in people do the four drugs work effectively together. And when you think about it, that makes sense, because the clinical trial was derived from the clinical results, and the model for VAMP was clinical leukemia, not mouse leukemia. It was in that setting that we knew about 6-MP and methotrexate, and the limit of toxicity, so we put it all together intellectually. But you see today we're living in a world where the intellect is gone, it's all empirical! Now you have to go to the FDA, and they say you can't do anything until you already know the answer. By their thesis you can't do anything original until you know it's going to work, and then of course it's not original!"

According to J, Zubrod also worried about the political consequences for NCI if Freireich's idea failed. "Zubrod had told Tom that we couldn't take a chance on doing something so experimental: if the children died, we'd be accused of experimenting on people at this federal installation at the National Cancer Institute. But Tom Frei thought it ought to be done and J Freireich wanted to do it and Zubrod wasn't going to stop us if we did it. Zubrod didn't give his approval, but he didn't interfere. I would have real trouble doing that myself. If one of my guys wanted to do something and I was totally opposed to it, I'd have trouble saying go ahead and feel free to do it. Particularly if it was dangerous. Yet everything new is dangerous. How can you discover anything unknown if you have to be sure that it isn't harmful? We could have killed all of those kids—no one could say in advance that we wouldn't.

"VAMP was especially emotional and exciting because we treated the patients one at a time. The first protocol I wrote was another kind of project that you couldn't do today. The VAMP protocol was written in what I call a Phase I–Phase II study. You build the requirement into the protocol that the doses and schedules are going to change as a result of the outcome of each patient study. (Technically it's called a Baysian statistical approach using continuous data analysis.) The VAMP protocol was written so that all the drugs were initially given by their full dose, with vincristine scheduled weekly, amethopterin (methotrexate) twice weekly, 6-MP daily orally, and prednisone daily orally.

"We treated thirteen children on this protocol, and by the time we got to the thirteenth, we knew the answer because we knew how to give the drugs. You can imagine the tension. I could just hear people saying, 'I told you so, this girl is going to die,' and 'The parents are going to complain that you experimented on her.' The key secret was really in the first patient. The doses we gave her were too high, and she almost died of toxicity. I sat with that first child, and God, she was so sick! We kept her going with antibiotics and respirators. I suppose I saw her eight times a day. Dr. Vince DeVita, who later became the director of the NCI, was a fellow with us then, and I used to drive him crazy because I was always hovering around. He'd say, 'Listen, I'm the doctor and I'll take care of the patient,' but these were my kids. I really tried to take care of them. I did little things, maybe I could make them more comfortable, give them a little aspirin, lower their temperatures, get them a blanket, or whatever. Anyway, she pulled through and ended up in a remission. (Later, sadly, the leukemia came back and she died.) We weren't discouraged by our initial awful experience in reaching that remission, and we decided we'd do it one more time. The second patient we worked with was Janice. This time we stopped the treatment at the right point, having learned from the first patient. When the bone marrow developed aplasia [absence of cells], that meant that we'd killed off all the cells and we needed to stop the treatment to allow the normal cells to recover. That's what we had not understood in the first patient. By not recognizing when to stop, the first patient got two extra days of chemotherapy and that was the thing that almost killed her. We knew better when we treated Janice in 1961, and in the late 1980s her picture appeared on the cover of *Cancer Research*, because she had been cured.

"The secret of our success was to treat intermittently and not continuously. We studied the data from our first two patients very carefully and decided that the time to give the drugs would be every ten days, and the third patient received VAMP for ten days as opposed to continuously. That turned out to be just right, and we never saw that kind of severe toxicity again. We got all the patients into remission, and the speed with which we got them into remission was so impressive it almost knocked us off our feet. It was faster than anything I've seen before, and there was no infection, no need for platelet transfusion, no nothing! It was another penicillin! Once we gave it for ten days and waited for the marrow to recover, 40 or 50 percent of our patients were in remission with just a single course of combination chemotherapy, and when we gave them a second course, almost all of them were in remission—only one child failed. And we said Wowee!

"We had entered these patients into our study one after the other, and we watched them very carefully. So we already had some of the kids in remission for a long time when the second important part of the VAMP study occurred to me. I thought, wow, this stuff is dynamite for inducing a remission. Maybe we should continue to use it in patients even after they are in a complete remission. That was a heretical notion at that time. By that point hematologists were convinced that chemotherapy could only keep the lid on the disease: you could never stop the treatment because, once you stopped, the children would invariably relapse. Moreover, you had to use very low doses of methotrexate and 6-MP because, the conventional wisdom said, if you gave the other drugs on a continuous basis, you would likely get into serious trouble. So we broke the prevailing concept of giving continuous low-dose treatment by treating the children aggressively even after all evidence of the leukemia was gone—I mean we treated with *full* doses. I'd like to take credit for having this idea, but it really belongs to my colleague, Dr. M. C. Li."

J and M. C. Li had known each other in Chicago, where they had been residents together. They came to the National Cancer Institute about the same time, and both of them found themselves in trouble for proposing and trying controversial new approaches to cancer treatment. Li, who was on the Endocrinology Service at NCI, was treating women who had a rare, wild-growing cancer of the uterus called choriocarcinoma. His success was based on a program of using high doses of methotrexate intermittently, long after the patients had seemingly returned to normal. Although the rest of the field took a long time to acknowledge it, Li's work marked the first time a widespread malignancy could be controlled and even cured by chemotherapy.

"Do you know that M.C., God bless him, may he rest in peace, got fired for claiming he could cure choriocarcinoma? I went over to his house for dinner, and we consoled one another. The unusual thing about chorio-carcinoma is that the cancer cells produce a very sensitive chemical marker, choriogonadotrophic hormone, the same substance that is normally ele-vated in pregnancy, and you can determine approximately how much cancer a person has by measuring the level of choriogonadotrophic hor-mone. When M.C. gave high doses of methotrexate, the tumor masses disappeared, the chest x-ray improved, and the patient looked normal; however, when he measured the hormone level, it was still abnormally high. M.C. figured the patient still had active carcinoma and needed more treatment, even though he couldn't find the tumor because it was so small. So he treated his patients intermittently with methotrexate until the hormone levels went down to zero. And that's what he got fired for, experimenting on people.

"M.C. was convinced that until you got the hormone down into the normal range, you shouldn't stop giving methotrexate. Of course M.C. was right: if you didn't treat them until the hormone levels were normal, the cancer invariably recurred and the patients died; if you did treat them, they were often cured, although Li didn't know that at the time. He had simply figured out that the hormone level was what you had to go by and not whether you could see the cancer cells when the tumor got very small. It seemed ridiculous. Everybody laughed at Li and the work hadn't been confirmed by anyone else, so M.C. was killed by the NCI. Zubrod tried very hard to protect him, but he couldn't. The director of the Cancer Institute, his immediate superior, the whole system at the Institute couldn't tolerate the man because he was so radical.

"I mean Li was really crazy; he was like Freireich! Imagine trying to cure choriocarcinoma, it's outrageous, you can't do that! It took the NCI about five years after M.C. was gone to make the claims that they'd cured widespread cancer and to confirm that he was right. They never admitted that it was Li who was responsible for that insight, but rather the credit went to other investigators who were there at the time. At least that is my opinion.

"But I saw the patients, and I saw the data and knew that M.C. was honest. I was impressed by that and I thought, my God, if VAMP can do what it's doing to get leukemia into remission, maybe we ought to continue to treat in the same way as M.C. did for choriocarcinoma even when there's no evidence of active leukemia and the patients are in remission.

"When Li left NCI, he went to Memorial Sloan-Kettering in New York and committed a second major crime, because he cured testicular cancer. You know what? He got fired again, the same way. He applied the same kind of reasoning to treating young men who had cancer of the testis that had spread throughout the body. Testicular cancer cells also produce hormone markers similar to choriocarcinoma. M.C. said that if you measure the hormones and find the levels are going up, then you have to treat with drugs because the cancer is advancing. When the levels go down, you keep on treating until the patient is cured, and that's how you cure testicular cancer! And they fired him from Memorial for treating people who were in remission, because everybody knew that you couldn't cure testicular cancer that way. These were very sick patients who all had very advanced cancer and a short life expectancy, and he was treating widespread testicular cancer, not just local disease. He made the claim that those patients could be cured, and that was outrageous; Memorial wouldn't stand for it. And after that, he went to a small hospital on Long Island where they let him set up a laboratory. Later he moved on to California and died of a stroke; he had hypertension.

"M.C. was the kind of person who makes America great. He came to the United States during the Chinese Communist Revolution. His brother had been a big mucky-muck with Chiang Kai-shek, and he couldn't get back into the country. His wife was in jail and his children were in jail, although they got out while M.C. was at NIH. This man was a giant. He cured cancer, the first widespread cancer [choriocarcinoma] to be cured in the world was done by this man. Happily that fact was recognized by giving him the Lasker Prize."

J Freireich's version of this little-known story differs from Jim Holland's (see Chapter 11) and those of other people. But the crucial point is the lively interplay of ideas among scientists at the National Cancer Institute. They were talking to each other, observing each other's patients, scrutinizing each other's data, and stretching each other's scientific horizons. Li's choriocarcinoma work provided the critical insight that you did not have to rely on standard means of detection like x-rays to tell if the tumor was still active—the sensitive hormone assay could guide your treatment. Leukemia had no such convenient chemical marker, but perhaps some of the same principles could be followed.

Indeed, under Zubrod's leadership, J and Frei and their colleagues had long been trying to measure leukemic activity as carefully as possible by counting bone marrow cells meticulously and relating those numbers to the doses of drugs they had administered. With methotrexate, the program was to induce remission by giving 2.5 milligrams of methotrexate a day until either the bone marrow cells disappeared or the patient went into remission. Then the dose would be lowered. To maintain the remission, much lower doses were given. The VAMP program had followed the same plan. But now Freireich wondered what would happen if he applied Li's idea to leukemia chemotherapy with VAMP. Could it cure his patients?

"I went to Tom with that idea and he said, like he always did, 'It sounds pretty good, J, I'll let you know.' Tom always wanted to do something a little more systematic, so he suggested that we double the low maintenance dose, or something like that. But I was adamant, because I thought we had to induce remission and keep on giving them that same high dose.

"Tom knew I wouldn't compromise, but he didn't like my idea. Now he's not like me—he's intellectual; when he got frustrated, he realized that he had to gather some additional information and that was really the start of cell kinetics [understanding the timing of cell division]. He had heard Zubrod and Howard Skipper talk about working in the mouse model, measuring the number of cells that had to be killed in order to cure leukemia [see Chapter 10]. Of course we were doing a similar thing in people, but it didn't dawn on him that we were doing it the other way around. We really knew what we had to do to cure leukemia. But Tom wanted to do a little thinking about it. So he and one of his fellows went to the pathology laboratory, with our friend Dr. Lou Thomas. They got the organs from the freezer of all of the children who had died of leukemia—there had been ten or twelve. They did the so-called Chalkley counts to determine how many leukemic cells there were per gram of spleen, liver, and kidney, measured the total weight of those organs, and did some arithmetic.

"Tom calculated how many leukemic cells there were in each organ and made some estimates as to how many there were in the total body. And then we went to Skipper and made some more calculations. Basically we figured that children didn't die of leukemia until they had 10^{12} [a trillion] leukemic cells in the body, or some similar number. Then Tom had to know how quickly the leukemic cells divided. We sat down with Dr. George Brecher and reviewed the bone marrow tests that we used to do every two weeks on the kids, and we counted the number of leukemic cells. We calculated that the number of mouse cells doubled about every four days. We constructed a mathematical model for humans, based on the prototype of the L_{1210} mouse model, and asked the question: Was it possible to cure leukemia? Those calculations described the kinetics of how rapidly cells divided and how rapidly they could be killed by our treatment. That way we carefully constructed a theoretical basis for curing children with leukemia.

"We'd had all of this experience with using single drugs before, and we knew that vincristine alone would put patients into remission in about six weeks and that their remissions would last for so many weeks. Similarly, we knew how long prednisone remissions lasted, and so on. So we took all of our data on the use of single agents—knowing that prednisone killed so many cells, full-dose vincristine killed so many cells, and combinations of 6-MP and methotrexate killed so many cells on the average—and we predicted that if we gave them together to patients in remission, that we'd kill so many cells and how long the remission would last. Then we predicted that if you gave another course of VAMP and achieved an equal cell kill, it would take so long for a relapse to occur, if it ever did. We calculated that three courses of VAMP could cure the patient, and we published these reviews and our predictions. The simple cell count method became the intellectual basis for the research to cure leukemia.

"A young colleague, Dr. Myron Karon, who was doing some psychological studies on our patients, persuaded us that the older children being studied really had to be involved in the decisions about them. Remember that some of our children were ten, twelve, or fifteen years old. So when a child was treated with VAMP and achieved remission, we sat down with the parents and child. We explained that the child was in remission, but that we had treated X number of people in the past and they all relapsed eventually. We further explained our notion that, if we treated such children aggressively they might die of toxicity from the drug, but on the other hand, we might cure them. We just couldn't know until we did it. If we didn't treat them aggressively, however, we knew the disease invariably came back and the children would die for sure.

"That was our hypothesis, based on the kinetics and on the previous experience with other drug programs. We thought they would all relapse unless we did something bold like VAMP. Well, the parents of the first child agreed and the parents of all of the other children agreed, as did the children. I never had a patient refuse experimental treatment at the National Institutes of Health: in my entire career, I've treated somewhere over 1,000 patients with acute leukemia, but I doubt I've had 10 patients refuse experimental treatment in all. (I still have the data on all 1,040 patients that I've treated up to this point, so when I publish my results I'm reporting on the full 1,040.)

"So the first parents agreed to let us take their now-healthy child who was in complete remission and bring him back into the hospital for another course of VAMP. We did this and the child became sick as hell and so did the subsequent ones, but nobody came close to dying. In fact, it was reasonably mild treatment compared to today's standards.

"The next stroke of genius I had made the tension and emotion run even stronger. I reasoned that, whether or not we cured these children, we must find out for their benefit and for the benefit of mankind how long it would take for them to relapse, or whether they really were cured following three courses of VAMP treatment after their initial remission. How can you find that out unless you stop the treatment thereafter? We needed that data on the cell growth kinetics: if we hadn't cured the children, the amount of time it would take for the leukemia to come back would tell us how many leukemic cells remained at the end of treatment.

"But the thought of stopping the treatment was just as traumatic as the thought of continuing to treat. Every day the parents would come and say, 'Dr. Freireich, my child is going to die of leukemia if you don't give him those drugs.' And I'd say, 'I know the drugs are going to work again, even if the patients relapse. I think they might be cured, but we can't find out if we don't do it. You're the first pioneers, and we're going to do it.' The tension was enormous. Zubrod made a point of coming on rounds every week, and the fellows thought I was insane. My young colleague Dr. Gerry Bodey went to his minister because he was so upset about the experiments we were doing on these children. But if you think it was tense when we started, imagine what happened when the first child relapsed after we stopped the treatment. Everybody said, 'Oh, my God, this is foolish. We better stop torturing people.' They wanted to go back to the simple maintenance program and all that. But I said absolutely not. Although one relapsed, I knew we still had others, and one is only one. But then a second one relapsed, and it was two out of whatever the number was of the group. However, we still couldn't be sure. By the time three patients relapsed, we threw in the sponge and thought it was all over. The children we were treating with three additional courses were mixed in with the children who relapsed and were coming back for additional treatment. The parents had a meeting, and there was just too much tension for everyone, so we stopped the whole thing. The children who relapsed were then successfully brought into remission with vincristine and prednisone. But we elected not to add any treatment for the children who were in remission until they did relapse. We pursued the study as it was originally designed, but stopped putting new patients into the study."

Why did this program fail, and what should they do next? Everything had been worked out so carefully in advance that there seemed to be no reason for its failure, but of course there had to be some reason. Tom and J went back to the drawing board. They were concerned by the fact that they didn't know whether or not giving four drugs at the same time was causing unfavorable drug interactions. Would the drugs antagonize each other and possibly even nullify their effects? Theoretically, at least, this was a possible reason for the program's failure.

The obvious solution was to go back to sequences: to give the same four drugs one after the other, each in full dose. Even if the patient's leukemic cells were not particularly sensitive to the full dose of a single agent, some leukemic cells would be killed, and then the next agent might kill some of the remaining cells, and so on. The basic notion was that if they gave the drugs as single agents one after the other, it might be more effective than if they gave them together. This program was called BIKE. In effect, it used vincristine and prednisone together to get the patients into remission. Next they administered a full dose of methotrexate, followed by a full dose of 6-MP, and then resumed the vincristine and prednisone. Because they gave two cycles of that sequence after remission was achieved, they dubbed the new treatment program *bi-cycle*: BIKE for short.

The BIKE program took four to six months to complete, which was a little longer than the VAMP treatment program. The courses were shorter because patients were treated for five days instead of ten, since the researchers knew the optimal doses for short courses. M. C. Li had used five equal day courses of methotrexate in treating choriocarcinoma. Freireich and his colleagues were also influenced by the time that it took for human leukemic cells to divide. It was important that the course of treatment attack at least two average cell divisions, so that if the drugs missed reaching cells part of the way through the process of cell division, they could get them the next time around.

Even as they got into the BIKE study, the children who had been treated previously with the VAMP regimen were beginning to shape up. These VAMP cases were not continued on treatment once they were in remission; yet it turned out that they stayed in remission as long as other patients who had been treated with continuous low-dose chemotherapy (that is, 6-MP) after entering remission. In both cases it was an average of thirty to thirty-two weeks before a relapse occurred. And in both cases, the average number of weeks before relapse was far longer than it was for patients who had not had either intensive combination chemotherapy or maintenance chemotherapy. This was a very important development. It meant that VAMP had done it—it had worked. But as these results were coming in, J and Tom were already embarked on the new BIKE study. They reasoned that the only problem with the VAMP treatment strategy was that the amount of chemotherapy given after the patient was in remission simply wasn't adequate.

"We were able to go from 10^9 [a billion] leukemic cells down to 10^6

[a million] or 10^3 [a thousand], but we didn't get to wipe out every last leukemic cell—which you have to do to be sure that you get a cure. We learned from the BIKE study that if you give the same drugs in sequence for a little bit longer, the patients stay in remission a little bit longer. In order to get more cell kill, it was going to be necessary to combine the BIKE and VAMP programs. We planned to give VAMP in five-day courses at higher doses and more often. We made estimates of how many leukemic cells remained in the children who had relapsed, based on the time that it took for the relapse to occur. [They were drawing on Howard Skipper's arguments about mouse leukemia—see Chapter 10.] We estimated that it would take the average child eight months, or about thirty-two weeks, to relapse. Allowing for a very rough error rate of ± 100 percent, we realized it might be necessary to treat the patients for a year in order to completely knock out their leukemic cells.

"Consequently the next study, our famous POMP [prednisone, vincristine (Oncovin), Methotrexate, 6-MP (Purinethol)] study, gave five-day courses of the same drugs every two weeks for a year. Oh boy! By the middle of the study it was going brilliantly, and the results were better than anything anyone had imagined in terms of remission duration. Of course we didn't yet have any long-term survival data, because we were only in the first year of the study. (The median duration of remission in the POMP-treated patients would turn out to be eighteen to twenty-four months, compared with six to seven months in the VAMP study.) But we knew that we had very few relapses and that the children were staying in remission, so we were clearly headed in the right direction. It was right in the middle of that study that Tom Frei resigned and moved to Houston.

"The situation was a real disaster for me! The POMP study had come to the point where we were going to need a hundred patients, not ten, because the study was so good, and here Frei up and decides to go to M. D. Anderson. The director wouldn't give us any more beds at NCI, nor could Zubrod. I wanted to use the cooperative groups to study the protocol, but they didn't want to mess with me and I was frustrated. Dr. R. Lee Clark, the president of M. D. Anderson, recruited me by saying that they then had two hundred beds just for patients with cancer, and they were going to add a five-hundred-bed hospital. He told me that I would be able to do anything I wanted and that the whole state of Texas would send us leukemia patients! In the meantime Tom's successor at NCI, Dr. Seymour Perry, said he wanted to stop the POMP studies and that he wanted me to leave. 'OK,' I said, 'but, if I leave, what are you going to do?' He told me he was going to appoint Dr. Ed Henderson, who had been a fellow of mine earlier on. Dr. Henderson and I made a deal. I said that I couldn't go to my grave unless I knew the answer to the POMP study. If it cured 50 percent of the children and we didn't know that because we didn't finish the study, it would be the greatest crime ever committed against nature. So we agreed that there would be no new patients registered into the POMP study, but they would complete it exactly as I had written the protocol, with twelve months of POMP treatment. Ed Henderson carried through and was senior author on the paper describing the study. My part of the agreement was that I would just leave and they would get all the credit; I wouldn't have anything to do with it, and I lived up to that. Henderson was wonderful, and just like one of my own family, a really super guy. [Dr. Henderson later moved to Roswell Park Memorial Cancer Institute, where he became chief of the Medical Service.] At that point I left NCI for M. D. Anderson Hospital, where I've been ever since."

As J Freireich looks back on his lifetime in leukemia research, his enthusiasm for his work is as intense as ever. Heart surgery has not slowed him down noticeably, and Deanie still has reason to complain that he puts work before family.

"Whenever she says that, I always agree with her, because it's only said when we are angry and having a disagreement about something or other. If I put my work above my family, I feel guilty, because you should put your family, your wife, your mother ahead of other humans. There are biblical and ethical bases for doing that. But the guilt doesn't last very long. I have been very lucky in being able to discover things. The satisfaction of being able to discover things outweighs whatever else I can do that makes me happy; you know, like eat, drink, sleep or be loved or get married or whatever.

"The joy of discovery seems to me the highest human experience. To know something that no one ever knew before you, is really something! And if they knew it before you and you didn't know they knew it, even that's extremely pleasurable. The joy of discovery is unsurpassable. One time I was asked to write a sentence for *Who's Who*, summing up my philosophy, and that sentence went something like this, 'To be able to contribute to the human condition knowledge which alleviates suffering and prolongs life, forever must be man's highest calling.' I feel so lucky to be able to do this kind of work, because what I can accomplish belongs to our species forever. No one can take it away, people like Hitler can't burn it, and if you cure a disease it's cured forever. M. C. Li cured choriocarcinoma; that isn't going to change forever, ever, ever. It makes you feel immortal in the real sense. We can only do the best we can with what we have in our lives, but the creative people live forever. And medical science does even more than live forever because it creates life. It's like being a mother in a gigantic sense. What if the 500,000 people who die of cancer in the United States every year didn't die; how many people can do that?"

J's impatience with nay-sayers remains unquenched. He still vividly recalls his fury in the 1950s when Dr. Sidney Farber said in public that "it was nice for young people to keep trying, but no one was going to cure leukemia with methotrexate, 6-MP, and prednisone; it was out of the question."

A decade later, he had mellowed enough—or was secure enough in his triumphs—to listen when Dr. Farber advised him that "it's very nice to talk about curing leukemia, but I really think you should moderate that view. Why don't you discuss it as 'prolonging life'?" Indeed, J said, "from 1965 on, I stopped using the word *cure* in my medical publications. And Farber—who didn't tell you something he had not thought about deeply— had proven to be at least partially right in the sense that even if we cure the leukemia or the cancer, the events that caused it may still be present and the individual is more prone to get it again. I've had patients who have 'relapsed' after ten years without treatment, and you can't convince me that it was really a relapse rather than a new leukemia. I think people who have had cancer are always at higher risk for getting it again, and there's perhaps no way to reverse that.

"But when I talk to lay people, I do use the word *cure*, because there's no dictionary that tells you what *cure* means in scientific terms. Does it mean five years disease-free? Does it mean that, if you die at age sixty or seventy-five of old age, that you've been cured, that for all those years after treatment you did not have leukemia? Maybe you still do have it, or the tendency to have it. We just don't know for sure.

"But people still think I'm kidding if I say I want to cure cancer. They laugh at me because they think it's a bloody joke. But I believe that cancer is the most important problem in therapeutic research, and leukemia is the most important problem in cancer. The way medicine is moving, heart disease is going to be largely gone in fifty years, and in a generation or two there won't be much problem with heart disease. So the cardiovascular problem is largely solved, and the people in that field will be out ditch digging. Cancer is the problem in biology, and people are still sitting around arguing about whether we've cured it or can cure it. That's all a bunch of bullshit; this is biology. We're talking about growth, proliferation of cells, differentiation of cells, and what are they arguing about?

"I believe that if we cure adult leukemia, we're going to cure cancer, because leukemia is the leading edge of cancer research. That's where the oncogenes are to be found, that's where the molecular genetics are, that's where the work with biological response modifiers is going on, that's where everything is. Why? Because the cells are right there in front of us. We can get pure cancer cells or leukemia cells every day of the week, and you can experiment with that in the laboratory. You did that, John, when you were here at the National Cancer Institute and started up the use of human leukemic cells in laboratory research. People can't do that with breast or lung cancer, and so you have to be frustrated if you want to work on those diseases. Forget about it until we understand it further. When we find something that's more effective in leukemia, then we have the chance to translate it to the other kinds of cancer. That's where the action is."

CHAPTER 9

Emil (Tom) Frei III, M.D.

*Do ye hear the children weeping, O my
   brothers,
Ere the sorrow comes with years?*
—*Elizabeth Barrett Browning*

When I first came to the National Cancer Institute in 1956 as a clinical associate, Dr. Frei was chief of the Leukemia Section in the Medicine Branch, and I worked on his service. Our first meeting was memorable for me; a quiet Sunday morning when Tom's children and their friends sprinted down the hallway of the laboratory part of the twelfth floor of the Clinical Center and jumped up to grasp the brass rings suspended from the ceiling. When the sprinklers activated, their squeals of delight turned to sheer terror. Tom remained calm, as though this were a regular occurrence.

Creativity takes many forms: Emil (Tom) Frei III grew up surrounded by artists and musicians, and his parents certainly expected him to be an artist of some kind, not a creative scientist. His grandfather had started the Emil Frei Art Glass Company in St. Louis. The business, which specialized in the design and making of stained-glass windows, was carried on by Tom's father, who was widely recognized for his adaptations of modern art to the stained-glass medium. Tom's brother Bob, and later his nephew Steve, headed the family business. His mother was a musician. The house was always full of artists and musicians, books and lively talk.

   "I chose my parents well. My mother was a concert pianist and the music reporter for the local St. Louis paper. My earliest memory is of sitting beside her at the piano, when she played or practiced. Starting in early grade school, I was permitted to leave Wednesday afternoons with my mother to go to the symphony. This was much more fun than school. But going to the symphony in grade school, at least in my grade school, labeled you as a sissy, and I often had to fend off the big boys Thursday morning as a price for that Wednesday afternoon.

"Music and Catholicism were not separate from each other or from our lives. They were intrinsic. I was recruited into the local church choir in the first grade and remained there until my voice changed. I can still sing many of the religious holiday church songs in Latin. But we could be bad boys as well. One sleepy, summer Sunday morning at five o'clock mass, we assembled in the choir around the organ. There were not more than twenty parishioners in the church. The priest was singing the Latin chant 'Dominus vobiscum,' to which we would respond 'Ora pro nobis.' But when we took over chant and response half the choir would sing, 'Whatd'ja have for breakfast?' while the other half would respond, 'Old rotten doughnuts.'

"Then, 'What's that between your teeth?' "

" 'Old rotten doughnuts.' "

"The priest, Father Mueller, stopped dead in his tracks on the altar, and his head turned to the choir. Of course the boys quickly returned to Latin. He shook his head. The choirmaster, a Mr. Dohm, while he never did find the culprits, announced that the making of a mockery of the religious ceremony was a mortal sin, punishable by hellfire.

"And there were other moments of comedy—sometimes ribald. During the Depression stained-glass windows were not selling well. My dad bid on a contract to make windows for the new cathedral in St. Louis in 1933 and was one of three finalists. Following Dad's selection as the winner, but before the contract was signed, Dad and Mom invited the archbishop and a priest to dinner. The big event arrived. The house and table were beautiful and we, my brother Bobby and I, were told to be on our best behavior. I was ten and Bobby was eight—not an age and sex that is compatible with good behavior. The meal was sumptuous, the wine delicious, the conversation lively—all was well. A few jokes were told, when Bobby raised his hand.

" 'I know a good joke.'

" 'What's that?" said the priest.

"A look of anxiety on my mother's face. 'It's all right, Mommy, it's a religious joke.' More anxiety on the part of my parents, but there was no way to stop it.

" 'Which stretches the furthest, rubber or skin?'

" 'I'll bite—rubber,' said the archbishop.

" 'Nope—it's skin,' said Bobby.

" 'How's that?'

" 'Because the Bible says that Moses tied his ass to a tree and walked five miles.' Dead silence. My parents saw the contract going down the tube. A guffaw from the archbishop and then from the priest—followed by great laughter. Dad got the contract. Bobby was disciplined with attenuation. He may have kept us in groceries during several years in the early years of the Depression."

Later in the 1930s the family found frugal ways to entertain itself: book discussion groups, play readings, field trips on a shoestring budget around St. Louis, square dancing, summer vacations at a family camp run by the Consumers Co-operative movement. As devout Catholics, religion played a big part in the Freis' lives. Tom's religious consciousness was directed more toward the beauty of the Church's art and music than toward doctrine. His choice of career and approach to medicine, however, were deeply influenced by the values of compassion and hope he took from his Catholic upbringing.

"As time passed and I became increasingly impressed by the fundamental truth and power of science, my faith receded, but was restored, at least in part, by the ecumenism of Pope John XXIII. I still enjoy immensely the holiday rituals with music."

The home was full of love and mutual respect, which provided the children with an enormous sense of security. Tom's father had great hope that he would go into the stained-glass window art and business. But he never showed it. When Tom announced his irreversible decision to go into medicine and science, his father was supportive and advised his son to "pick a big problem and stay with it."

Although Tom enjoyed art and music at home, the subjects that affected him the most were mathematics and the sciences, particularly physics. A Jesuit, Father Benoit, who was his teacher in the first year of high school, had a great love for these subjects and became a close friend. The fundamental and often sudden insights that occur in algebra, geometry, and later in calculus gave him a sense of the joy and power of science. Biology at the time was largely descriptive and taxonomic. "Recently I had occasion to pull out my old high school biology book of about 1938. If you have any questions about the total revolution that has occurred in science, just compare that book with a modern biology book."

The book that probably had the greatest influence on his choice of medicine as a career was the classic book on epidemiology, *Rats, Lice, and History*, by Hans Zinsser. The Zinsser book brought together good science, careful observation, a sense of history, adventure—and also a sense of danger—which always appealed to Tom. Also inspiring was *Man the Unknown*, by Alexis Carrel, a French physician-scientist who had worked with Charles Lindbergh (a part of Lindbergh's life not many people know about) for a year in Paris. They cultured living cells taken from a chicken heart and were able to get cell lines growing that persisted for many years in the laboratory. *Man the Unknown* was a speculative story, almost science fiction, about how humans would evolve in the coming hundreds of years. "That influenced me in the direction of medicine and away from straight mathematics and physics."

In 1941 Tom started off at St. Louis University as an art student, as his parents had hoped. But in his second year, when he turned eighteen and had to register for the draft in the midst of World War II, Tom decided to sign up for the premedical program. He was summoned for active duty in the summer of 1943 and was sent by the navy to Colgate University for premedical courses. It was as simple as that: "The direction of my career, the decision between science and medicine on one hand versus art on the other was determined by those circumstances. I probably would have gone that way in any case, but it's not certain."

The transition from the highly disciplined parochial schools and Jesuit university to the secular Colgate was exciting, despite the strenuous educational schedule the military premedical program required. The trainees got up at 5:30 in the morning, jogged, marched, did their military training, had breakfast, and then started classes at 8:00 A.M. They had examinations and evaluations at every turn.

Because of the war, the program was accelerated, putting aside the humanities and stressing the sciences. Tom took three years' worth of academic work in two calendar years. Out of his class of 150 pre-meds, Tom was one of the handful accepted immediately into medical school. He never formally took his bachelor's degree; he just went straight on to Yale Medical School.

Yale was just the right medical school for young Tom. It had a small class, forty-eight, and hardly anyone was married. Few had cars, so that the students were thrown together in intimacy for four years. Yale offered no compulsory examination except for National Board Examinations at the end of the second and the fourth year. This was done to encourage students to individualize their curriculum, with emphasis on academia and research. Lack of compulsory examinations also took away some of the anxiety and confrontational aspects of medical school, which can be very intense for budding young doctors. Like many European schools, Yale required a thesis to achieve an M.D. Tom dabbled in a number of projects, finally fixing on microbiology and the pathogenesis of the chronic, infectious lung disease known as bronchiectasis. To learn to do advanced independent study serves every professional well, almost regardless of the topic that is being researched.

"The dormitory in which I lived during most of medical school was right next to the Yale nurses' dorm, Nathan Smith Hall. That kind of juxtaposition of young men and women working in the same profession, at an age when hormone titers are riding high, can lead to marvelous interactions. This was the mid-forties and, compared with today, it was still an age of innocence. We would often go out as a group to a party or dance. In my third year, I fell in love with a beautiful, strong-willed nurse by the name of Liz, who later became my wife and the mother of my children."

They married in New Haven.

After an internship at St. Louis University, Tom went briefly into medical practice in Oklahoma to support his young family. When the Korean War broke out, Tom was drafted back into the navy and spent a year as the only medical officer for a destroyer squadron of 2,500 men in the Pacific and Far East. Tom quickly learned a lot about medicine: parasitic diseases, venereal diseases, wounds, respiratory disease, and psychiatry.

Tom used the time in the navy to continue studying medicine; he yearned to go into academic medical research. His chance came in January 1953 when he got out of the military and took a residency, first at Washington University in St. Louis and then, when a full-time Hopkins group moved to St. Louis University, at his alma mater.

An outstanding group of medical academics had been recruited from Hopkins. This included the chairman of the Department of Medicine, Dr. Phillip Tumulty, and Dr. Gordon Zubrod, who was an associate professor. They brought commitment and excellence to the teaching of clinical medicine with an emphasis on the mechanisms (pathobiology) of disease. This had made Hopkins the first great medical school in the United States. Both the science and the art of medicine were emphasized. As a resident in medicine Tom showed an interest in research, and, in what would be an important relationship to both of them in the future, Dr. Zubrod took him under his wing. A newly discovered microorganism, then known as the pleuro-pneumonia-like organism, was thought to be causative in certain types of respiratory infections. Tom and his mentor worked out a technique of causing an infection in the external ear canal of the rat by direct injection of the organisms. They defined the natural history of that infection and its prevention and cure by antibiotics. Indeed, the then-new antibiotic tetracycline turned out to be highly effective. This experience taught Tom about the power of the laboratory in addressing clinical problems. The clinical investigator must be capable of bringing science to hypotheses that are generated at the bedside. Often the science will require that the doctor take the problem to the laboratory and work it out in simple, more definable systems before it's taken back to the bedside.

In addition, during that year and a half with Dr. Zubrod, Tom conducted a randomized comparative study of tetracycline versus penicillin in the treatment of pneumococcal pneumonia. This immersed him in the experimental design, conduct, and analysis of clinical trials, something that was to stand him in good stead later on at the National Cancer Institute. There was no formal training in research methodology for medical scientists; this was as close as one could get at that time. It was a great joy and source of pride that his first paper was accepted by, and published in, the prestigious *New England Journal of Medicine*.

"Like all research, there was a light side. I had to observe the rats and feed them frequently. I would take two cages home over the weekend and hide them on a high shelf in the basement. But my children discovered them and, unbeknownst to me, two rats escaped in the basement late one Saturday afternoon. That evening, we had a cocktail party for couples in the neighborhood. I heard this terrified scream from one of the wives, who had discovered one of the rats on the loose in the basement. The party became chaotic as several of us managed, after about an hour, to capture the two rats. My children were absolutely delighted."

After Zubrod left St. Louis and joined the brand-new National Cancer Institute, he recruited his young protégé, Tom Frei. "Gordon was not recruited to NCI because he was an oncologist—God knows there were virtually no oncologists at the time. Gordon told me about the new Clinical Center at NCI, a great new research building that had been opened in

1953. He told me this was an opportunity to enter a new era—to be in on the ground floor of understanding cancer and treating cancer with chemotherapy."

Up until then, Tom had not been responsible for the medical care of children, except for the practical experience his rapidly growing family (five children in all) gave him. And he knew very little about cancer. Unfortunately, the conventional medical wisdom was that doctors could do nothing for cancer patients beyond controlling their pain. The few cancer patients he had cared for confirmed the textbooks. In looking back on those days, Tom observed: "If that's your approach to patients, then it is hard to make a close identification with them when you make ward rounds. You tend to see the patients with enthusiasm if you think you can help them. But if you know you're not going to do much more beyond making the diagnosis, and you know they are going to go downhill rapidly and die, then you really don't generate much enthusiasm. But the real challenge in life generally, and in the care of patients particularly, is not what you do when you succeed, but what you do when you do not succeed. There were few successes in the treatment of disseminated cancer in 1955. It was usually a matter of watching the tumor get bigger, and the patient, progressively smaller. That was the challenge—the real test of a physician. My father's advice to me as a young man was to tackle a big problem and stay with it. I was totally committed to the position that science could solve the cancer problem."

Most of the people Tom consulted about NCI advised him to get an advanced degree in biochemistry, not to go directly into research on cancer treatment. They thought that was a guaranteed dead end to his hopes for a career in medical research. First master the basic science, he was told, then apply it to a clinical discipline. This was certainly sound advice for that time. But Zubrod's minority opinion carried the day. Tom was persuaded by Zubrod's argument that if you were a clinician, it made more sense to identify a research area and a clinical problem within it, and then marshal all the resources you could.

In February of 1955, with his wife, Elizabeth, and four children, Mary, Emil, Alice, and Nancy, ages six to two, Tom drove their old beat-up Studebaker from St. Louis to the Pennsylvania Turnpike, dropped down to Rockville Pike and then Wisconsin Avenue in Bethesda, and turned in at the sign that said National Institutes of Health. Even before going to the house where they were to stay, Tom stopped at the huge brick structure on the hill, the Clinical Center, went into the large lobby, and had his first look at what was to be his professional home for the next ten years.

When Tom arrived at NIH at the tender age of thirty-one, the Clinical Center had not been open for too long. Half the patient rooms were empty, and half the laboratory space unoccupied. The resources available for research were unparalleled: patients; space; equipment; bright, dedicated colleagues. The Clinical Center had laboratories and patient care areas closely integrated in space and organization so as to maximize the opportunity to integrate laboratory research into the clinic. He was in the right place at the right time—"We were very lucky!"

Tom decided to focus his research on the treatment of leukemia. In contrast to many university medical centers, NIH physicians and scientists led protected lives, professionally. They did not have to teach, committee work was minimal, they did not have to write grants, and the administrative/fiscal aspects of patient care were thoroughly covered by others. That was the good news.

The bad news was that if you were a new clinical investigator interested in therapeutic research, where did you start? The science of biomedicine was still primitive by today's standards. Even so, there were scientists at NCI who had developed tissue culture techniques for leukemia cells, and others who transplanted leukemias in mice. And the discovery of the structure of DNA by Watson and Crick in 1953 had provided a profound stimulus and frame of reference for basic science. Many of the biochemists at NIH were working in the new field of molecular biology, which would later revolutionize our understanding of how cells divide and control their functions.

But almost all of this was still in the future. In 1955 scientists occasionally talked about molecules, such as chemotherapeutic agents, and their targets, such as the enzyme dihydrofolate reductase for methotrexate. The theory of antimetabolites had been developed, but chemotherapy for cancer was the new kid on the block compared with long-established treatments such as surgery and radiotherapy. "The fact that there were several agents that were effective in the treatment of acute leukemia, that the beginnings of the science for a cancer drug development existed, and that models for the study of leukemia and tissue culture in animals were developed led us to select acute leukemia for our focus of therapeutic research. Dr. Zubrod had the major hand in that decision. Jim Holland, who preceded me at NCI, had also begun to focus on acute leukemia."

Given that decision during his first several months at NCI, Tom spent essentially all of his time learning about clinical and experimental leukemia. Experimentally, leukemia could be transplanted within inbred strains of mice. This made possible a number of quantitative therapeutic studies. Dr. Lloyd Law had produced methotrexate resistant L_{1210} leukemia cell lines. Using a test developed by the Nobel laureates Luria and Delbruck, Law demonstrated that resistant cells were already present at the time of treatment and were "selected out" by the treatment. Moreover, he found that resistance to one drug did not cross to another (methotrexate to mercaptopurine). Dr. Abe Goldin reasoned that lack of cross resistance was a rationale for combination chemotherapy. He demonstrated in this quantitative model that methotrexate and 6-MP were in fact synergistic when used in combination. He found that the dose of each agent profoundly affected response, for example, a linear increase in dose produced a log increase in tumor cells killed. He also found that the effectiveness of chemotherapy was much greater against a low as compared with a large cell number. Finally, new agents and new combinations could be tested and evaluated in this system, and then ranked quantitatively in terms of their therapeutic effect. All of these factors—dose, combinations, tumor numbers, drug resistance—would be central to Tom's clinical research through the next ten years—indeed, for the remainder of his career. These were exciting times at NCI.

But in the clinic, the situation for leukemia was totally different—indeed, almost polar. Prior to 1955, quantitative studies were lacking. For example, Tom was interested in knowing the relative response rates of agents like 6-MP and methotrexate. It was impossible. No one had defined response, which meant that everyone used different, often loosely stated criteria. It was not surprising, given this situation, that response rates varying from 0 to 60 percent were reported. Marrows during and/or following treatment were not obtained. Patients included in studies were poorly defined and often included, in addition to children with acute lymphocytic leukemia, patients with other forms of leukemia and lymphoma, and older patients. Response breakdown within certain disease and prognostic categories was not reported. Finally, the dose, schedule, and duration of treatment and other variables were not specified.

"Dr. Zubrod's major scientific contribution was his insistence on the development of quantitative prospective clinical trial designs. How could we determine in the qualitative chaos whether two drugs were better than one, whether platelets worked, indeed any research (and that's essentially all good research) that required quantitation." It has been said that research must begin with focus and quantitation. Tom was ideally poised to study and develop modern quantitative trial techniques to leukemia because of his previous training with Dr. Zubrod in the pneumonia trial during his residency.

Nineteen fifty-five was a watershed year. Major contributions had been made prior to that time. Indeed, demonstrating that methotrexate and 6-MP were active was important. But to build incrementally on such observations and to progress with certainty requires quantitation—in this case the prospective quantitative clinical trial. The introduction of such trials was essential to the marked acceleration in progress in the treatment of acute lymphocytic leukemia that was to come, for progress in cancer research, generally, and indeed, for all research.

Tom's job was made at once easier and harder by the arrival of Emil J Freireich in July 1955, only two months after his appointment as chief of the Leukemia Service. J was fresh from his hematology fellowship and full of cockiness from his Boston training. When J first came up and introduced himself as Emil Freireich, Tom could not believe his ears. "To get a job here, you don't have to assume that name," Tom told him.

Tom soon recognized Freireich's extraordinary, unique qualities. "J quickly became my closest professional friend and confidant. We talked two or three hours, mainly about research, almost every day for seventeen years. J's cardinal attribute was his creativity. He was capable of looking at problems from many different viewpoints, interpreting and analyzing them from his broad knowledge of both basic science and clinical science. The same broad-based experience provided a jumping-off ground for in-ductive development of novel approaches for research and treatment. His skills at communication, enthusiasm, and intelligence made it possible for him to present a new idea or approach with great vigor and effectiveness."

Tom and J shared strong personalities that commanded attention, and much of the creativity and progress of the chemotherapy-leukemia program derived from their interaction. The spirited interplay between Frei and Freireich comes through vividly in Tom's recollection of a conversation one evening, probably in 1961. Their discussion sticks in Tom's mind in part because it led to the crucial recognition that combinations of chemotherapeutic drugs, delivered in full doses as early as possible in the disease, would be the most successful way to treat leukemia: the basis of the VAMP treatment program for acute leukemia (see Chapter 8), MOPP for Hodgkin's disease, as well as combination drug therapies for other kinds of cancer. But he also remembers it because it was the only time he ever saw Freireich silenced. "J and I were having an animated conversation in my office. For some reason, I had received a glass top for my desk—probably the government had decreed that employees above a certain grade would get glass desk-tops. J's voice crescendoed with excitement at a new idea and, at the peak, he brought his fist down on the desk to emphasize his point. The glass shattered. For ten minutes, he was mute. Thus I was able to make my point without interruption, at the end of which we laughed together."

The biggest difference between the two young scientists lay in their approaches to dealing with their colleagues. "J was confrontational, controversial, and could be difficult." Watching J, Tom often wondered if the people most deeply involved in the creative process, "those who could see the distant shore more clearly than most," would almost, by definition, be controversial.

"Perhaps intrinsic to creativity is difficulty with authority. Throughout J's career he has had a confrontational and often difficult relationship with those in charge. While he worked in my section, my relationship to him was much more as colleague than as boss. But, nevertheless, it was not always a comfortable relationship. In addition, he intensely personalized and dramatized his research. There is certainly nothing wrong with this when the research is creative and productive, which it was. But J could present research in a way that antagonized major players in the field including, sometimes, his colleagues. This was bad enough if you were a collaborator, but particularly difficult if, in your view, it was your idea and you were the primary player. I don't believe this was deliberate but, rather, an expression of the emotional and personal intensity he brought to his research. On the other hand, J could be profoundly stimulating in scientific discussions and most ingratiating."

By virtue of both his position and his temperament (and Zubrod's exemplar as scientist-administrator), Tom was much more inclined to negotiate compromises that would enable the research to go forward. On at least one occasion—the joint IBM-NCI development of a machine for blood cell separation and transfusion (see Chapter 8)—it meant removing his friend as principal investigator because Freireich was "absolutely unwilling to compromise" with the other people involved on the project. "Yet our friendship survived this and many such episodes because of the positive side of the ledger: the progress in improving cancer treatment totally over-shadowed the problems. He was and remains my closest professional friend." This unwillingness to compromise is probably what cost J the most at NCI. For example, the IBM people did not wish to work with J but would accept collaboration with Dr. Perry—as Tom is aware.

The first and most obvious problem Tom faced in the management of children with acute lymphocytic leukemia was bleeding. Indeed, on his first visit to the four leukemia inpatients at the Clinical Center, two had ongoing hemorrhaging, one had an intermittent nosebleed, and the other one had bloody stools. Essentially, all of the patients had bleeding at some time, and the majority of patients died of, or with, major bleeding. Bleeding could occur into any site—the skin, the bowel, the eyes, the sputum, the brain. It was exceedingly morbid and frightening, as well as deadly. "The first thing I had to do was the classical approach to nosebleed, that is cauterizing and finally packing the front of the nose and leaving it in place. This was profoundly uncomfortable. It was often further magnified when a posterior [back of the nose] pack had to also be put in. Thus my first priority to research within a month of arriving was to study such hemorrhage."

Tom's careful review of fifteen patients seen at NCI since the opening of the Clinical Center in late 1953 clearly established that bleeding corre-lated with severe thrombocytopenia, a decrease in the number of blood platelets. Platelet transfusions had been given on some twenty occasions to these patients. However, this was generally done by transfusing one or two units of fresh blood, far short of the six platelet units that is generally the minimum given today. Nevertheless, in this retrospective study, there was a clear association between platelet transfusions and the temporary cessation of bleeding. Tom deduced that platelet transfusion would be a logical approach to the control of bleeding in acute leukemia. But research is not just a matter of what has to be done. The question is how. We heard earlier that the director of the blood bank and his supervisor, who was in charge of the Clinical Pathology Program, were reluctant and finally refused to provide platelets for two reasons: (1) patients would become immunized to platelets in a short period, after which they would no longer be effective; (2) such transfusions, even if they worked, would provide only a temporary respite because these patients were destined to die of their disease within a few months in any event.

"J Freireich, on his arrival, joined me in this study to provide ample fresh platelets to the site of blood vessel injury. The confrontation with the blood bank escalated and finally resulted in a large meeting in the auditorium addressed to the science and policy of platelets and platelet transfusions at the Clinical Center. I presented the retrospective study, indicating that platelets were effective. Most of the physician-scientists there, which included senior hematologists, probably believed that platelet transfusions would be effective but that the control of bleeding would be very short lived, an achievement which is questionable in dying patients. It was in this setting of turbulence that Zubrod came forward to speak and created, for me, what was a precious moment in the history of cancer research. In paraphrase, he said that the cure of acute leukemia might occur tomorrow, in the near future, in the distant future, or maybe never. If it was to be achieved, it would require multiple steps, that is, it would be incremental. He then said that one step that had to be taken was the control of hemorrhage. The most logical, immediate approach to this was to apply and to study platelet transfusions. He regarded it as his responsibility as clinical director of the NCI to see to it that this happened."

"I'd follow that man anywhere," Tom thought to himself.

Impasse. Clearly, they needed to demonstrate unequivocally the effectiveness of platelets. Tom, J, and Gordon got together after that meeting and decided to trot out the most powerful experimental design tool for clinical trials and apply it to platelet transfusions. They were in an ideal position to do this, because, as we shall see, they had developed quantitative clinical trial techniques for cancer chemotherapy. Thus they constructed a randomized comparative, double-blind study, the dramatic results of which were presented in Chapter 8. Indeed, the results of this study led to a major commitment on the part of NCI and, finally, even the blood bank to platelet acquisition facilities. The three-bag system for platelet collection was worked out by J and Alan Kliman in the blood bank. The inverse relationship between bleeding and platelet count was quantified. Platelet increments, as a result of transfusion dose, were established. The indications for platelet transfusions for the treatment and then for the prevention of hemorrhage were worked out. "This was a landmark contribution to cancer and hematology and continues to the present time to be a necessary, essential component of cancer chemotherapy and bone marrow transplantation. J deserves and gets the major credit for this achievement."

Perhaps the greatest overall contribution that Tom Frei made to the cure of childhood leukemia—and to cancer therapy generally—was his insistence on carrying out quantitative, prospectively designed, often randomized clinical trials. Before 1955 the clinical trials of new drugs and protocols for administering them were qualitative, often anecdotal, and usually inconclusive. The clinical trial of platelet transfusions to prevent bleeding is a case in point. Before 1955 researchers' opinions of the value of platelet transfusions—based on their experience and reading of the literature—ranged from effective, to transiently effective, to ineffective. Putting the question to a quantitative randomized comparative trial demonstrated the value of platelets decisively, and the whole field could move on to other problems. Science usually progresses incrementally through a series of questions (or, to put it more formally, hypotheses), but to move from one question to the next almost always requires a quantitative answer to the first question. It has been wisely said that science begins with the ability to count.

Before 1955 experiments with cancer therapy were haphazard. Often the reports would not define the patients' status clearly, ignored their prior treatment, and generally paid little attention to the many variables that affect response to chemotherapy. As we have seen, even the term *remission* meant different things to different researchers. With Dr. Zubrod's encouragement, Tom and J, with the continued involvement of Dr. Holland, set out to put cancer clinical trials on a genuinely scientific basis. They required each trial to have a precisely defined objective, a specified sample of patients (usually all very similar with respect to age, kind of leukemia, stage of disease, and other factors), a set treatment procedure, and well-defined measures of disease activity.

Some doctors felt that scientific clinical trials were counter to the best practice of medicine, because they limited the doctor's ability to tailor treatment to each patient individually. No two patients are the same and—felt these critics—no two should be treated identically. "These were and are legitimate concerns, and we took them very seriously. All patients were thoroughly informed and gave written consent. No treatment of established efficacy was withheld from the patient. The physician was enjoined not to follow the protocol in any circumstance where it was counter to the patient's best interest. Finally, patients could remove themselves from the protocol at any time. The doctor is a physician first, and scientist second. In my view, the two, science and medicine, are rarely in conflict. Indeed, the physician-scientist commitment in a given area is a plus for the patient in most respects. Research in experimental design continues as an ongoing process. While the nature of medical care delivery in the United States makes comparisons difficult, there is no evidence over the past forty years that the scientific clinical trial compromises the best patient care."

Detecting and measuring the patient's response to treatment was a particularly complex problem. Acute lymphocytic leukemia is primarily a disease of the bone marrow. Yet before 1955, response was judged by indirect criteria: blood changes, symptoms, changes in lymph nodes or spleen. Tom and his team found that examining the bone marrow itself was critical for gauging the effect of therapy. That meant doing frequent bone marrow aspirations and examinations. The only way they could be sure that a patient had reached complete remission was by looking at the bone marrow and seeing no leukemic cells at all and seeing a return of normal bone marrow cells. "In those first few months I can recall our amazement and enthusiasm as we gazed down the barrel of a microscope at a marrow that had been 100 percent replaced by leukemic cells four weeks before and which was now normal, that is, no identifiable leukemic cells. The joy that we felt when such a complete remission occurred in one of our patients in the mid-1950s was tempered by the fact that it didn't happen very often, and all patients relapsed." Their critics emphasized that the agents were toxic and that all patients were destined to die from their leukemia anyway. What should be the initial goal of treatment? They needed good methods and solid data.

No one knew whether, during a remission, there were still leukemic cells in the bone marrow, and if so, how many. With Zubrod's encouragement, Tom and J took the critical step of requiring regular bone marrow tests on *all* their patients, even those in a state of complete remission. The number of leukemic bone marrow cells was the best-defined measure of how sick, or well, a patient was. The use of the test forced Frei and his colleagues to define what they meant by remission—the phrase "complete remission" was, in fact, never used before 1955. Before then, doctors had simply said loosely that the patient was in a remission or that the patient was better. By "complete remission," the NCI researchers meant that the patient had no sign of the disease, had normal blood counts, felt healthy, and (like a normal person) had fewer than 5 percent immature blood cells, called blasts, in the bone marrow sample. A patient in complete remission could not be considered cured—at that point, no one could even hope for a complete cure—but would at least be able to enjoy weeks or months of normal, pain-free life out of the hospital.

Using their new criteria to define a complete remission and other quantitative definitions for a partial remission, the NCI team found that some of the drugs doctors thought were great were really not so good. When the two key antimetabolite drugs, 6-MP and methotrexate, were given as single agents, they only produced a complete remission rate only 10 to 30 percent of the time. The steroid prednisone produced a slightly higher rate.

In principle the usefulness of regular bone marrow tests should have been obvious, but parents and many doctors understandably resisted the idea of inflicting the pain of the test on such sick children. To some, it seemed terribly unfair to do periodic tests on a child who was in remission, behaving and feeling quite normal. The policy brought down plenty of criticism on Frei and Freireich, as the senior attending officers on the Leukemia Service, and on Zubrod, for authorizing the tests.

Tom, both as a doctor and as a father, had to sympathize with his critics. But the occasional recoveries—and the inevitable relapses—of his patients on the Leukemia Service deeply moved him. They spurred him to concentrate on the ultimate goal of bringing about complete remissions and prolonging them for everyone with leukemia.

At this juncture it is useful to review the sequence of chemotherapy protocols developed at NCI, which embodied the institute's major contributions to the cure of childhood leukemia. And who better to help with that than the chief of the Leukemia Service, Dr. Tom Frei. Furthermore, he was chairman of the Acute Leukemia Group B for the critical years 1955 through 1965. As we go through the studies we remind ourselves that these were the most successful ones—there were many others as well. The advances were always incremental when they occurred, leading to major insights, but step by step.

From 1955 to 1963, Tom Frei laid out the strategy for one clinical trial after another, coordinated the work of researchers in several hospitals, and keenly watched the patients under his own care as they went through the protocols. He continued to be an active participant in the trials after Dr. Holland took over as chair of Acute Leukemia Group B, and he himself moved from NCI to Houston. Between 1955 and 1968, the Acute Leukemia Group undertook ten different protocols that yielded positive important results. When Tom looks back at the work accomplished in these trials, he is quick to point out that, first, many other concurrent studies did not pan out; second, to find enough patients for this kind of quantitative research, a genuine collaboration among several institutions (initially NCI and Roswell Park in Buffalo, later St. Jude in Memphis and others) was essential; and third, while the research in these protocols got and deserved lots of credit, it depended on highly creative hypotheses generated in earlier, less visible phases of research that often went unrecognized.

The ten protocols summarized in the accompanying table are worth a close look—not just because of the increasing success of the treatments over the thirteen years, in hindsight, so striking, but also because the experiments and their interpretations reveal so much about the development of biomedical science.

In Protocol I (1955), Tom and his colleagues tried using two different antileukemic agents (6-MP and methotrexate), on two different schedules. The effort gave them their first taste of the issues involved in setting up and running a quantitative clinical trial. Methodologically, though, the study was flawed because they did not include control groups for each drug separately and because the actual treatment objective was not clear— were they trying to obtain some remission, a longer than average remission, or complete remission?

The critical insight from this protocol came as a by-product of their retrospective analysis of all the variables: they discovered that the most powerful determinant of survival was reaching complete remission. Because survival, particularly long-term survival, was the ultimate endpoint, this would indicate that the attainment of a complete remission was a logical and major short-term goal. Moreover, the prolonged survival in patients achieving a complete remission was largely due to time spent in complete remission, where the quality of life was good. Finally, since the marrow was the primary seat of the disease and generally contained the majority of the leukemia cells in the body, the extent of marrow infiltration reflected tumor cell kill and thus was a logical endpoint. At the onset of treatment, the initial marrow examination usually showed 100 percent

Landmark Clinical Trials

Protocol	Year started	Drugs and schedule of administration	Results	Comments
I	1955	All patients receive 6-MP plus daily or every 3 days MTX.	CRs are the most powerful determinants of survival.	First quantitative prospective experimental design for cancer treatment. Comparison of two groups was inconclusive.
II	1957	Patients randomized to MTX followed by 6-MP, 6-MP followed by MTX, or both together.	22% CR with MTX first. 28% CR with 6-MP first. 45% CR with both.	First definitive study of combination chemotherapy. Combined use was most effective.
III	1957	Actively bleeding patients randomized to receive fresh or bank blood transfusion (platelets vs. no platelets).	No platelets: 9% stopped bleeding. Platelets: 92% stopped.	Demonstration that fresh platelets control bleeding.
IV	1959	Prednisone to induce a CR, followed by randomization to (a) 6-MP during remission; (b) placebo during remission.	(a) 10-month CR. (b) 2-month CR.	First study of treatment for microscopic tumor. Set paradigm for chemotherapy with adjuvants during remission.
V	1961	Prednisone to induce CR, followed by randomization to (a) full dose of combined CPA, 6-MP, + MTX; or (b) half dose of combined CPA, 6-MP, + MTX.	(a) 15-month CR. (b) 6-month CR.	Demonstrates the importance of dose.
VI	1961	VCR + prednisone to induce CR, followed by randomization of MTX to (a) intermittent schedule (every 4 days); or (b) continuous daily MTX.	(a) 9-month CR. (b) 4-month CR.	Demonstrates importance of drug schedule in remission.
VII	1961	VCR + prednisone to induce CR, followed by randomization to (a) combination therapy daily 6-MP + MTX every 4 days or (b) single agent (6-MP or MTX) therapy.		Demonstration of superiority of combination chemotherapy in CR.
VIII	1962	VAMP	10–15% cure.	First study of intermittent, intensive combination chemotherapy.
IX	1963	VCR + prednisone to induce CR, followed by randomization to (a) 6-MP + MTX or (b) 6-MP + MTX + intrathecal MTX.	(a) 60% developed meningeal leukemia. (b) 20% developed meningeal leukemia.	First study of CNS prophylaxis with intrathecal MTX leading to decreased incidence in meningeal leukemia, but median survival was unchanged, despite some long-term survivors (10–15% cures).
X	1968	VCR + prednisone to induce CR, followed by randomization to (a) 6-MP + MTX; or (b) 6-MP + MTX + intrathecal MTX + CNS radiotherapy.	(a) No cures. (b) 35% cure.	Demonstration that chemotherapy plus radiation of brain markedly reduced the rate of meningeal leukemia and produced a 35% cure rate.
	1995	Modern multi-agent therapy.	75–80% cure.	Treatment now includes 7–8 agents. VAMP plus asparaginase, daunorubicin, cytosine arabinoside (or others).

NOTE: CR = complete remission; 6-MP = 6-mercaptopurine; MTX = methotrexate; CPA = cyclophosphamide; VCR = vincristine; VAMP = vincristine, aminopterin, 6-MP, prednisone.

infiltration with leukemia cells. Thus the complete elimination of identifiable leukemic cells from the marrow clearly represented a major antileukemic effect. The knowledge that achieving a complete remission was a legitimate short-term goal profoundly affected the mood and enthusiasm of the doctors and nurses participating in the program. When a complete remission was achieved, this knowledge and enthusiasm played back to the patient and their family.

For Tom and J, the attainment of the complete remission as a first goal of treatment became and has remained a principle in therapeutic research in cancer. Indeed, for almost all tumor types, the achievement of an initial complete remission is associated with a marked improvement in survival rate and is the first and essential step to cure.

Unfortunately, complete remissions were achieved in relatively few patients at first. The next step was to increase the complete remission (CR) rate, that is, the proportion of patients who achieved a CR. Protocol I had produced an overall 38 percent complete remission rate.

In 1957 the Acute Leukemia Group corrected the methodological problems of the first protocol by doing the necessary comparisons between combinations of drugs and the same drugs used alone. Protocol II was, in fact, the first definitive study of combination chemotherapy and is now regarded as a classic clinical experiment. The combination of 6-MP and methotrexate was somewhat, but not impressively, superior to the individual agents. The study also allowed the researchers to see whether the order of administering the drugs made a difference. The results proved hard to analyze, however, because so many patients in the study died from the disease before they could reach the second phase of treatment. Protocol III was the study that put platelet transfusion on the map as the way to control bleeding.

In Protocols IV–VI, the trials demonstrated that remission rates for single drugs ranged from 21 percent to 50 percent, but that combinations of two or more drugs with complementary toxicities could produce much higher remission rates. The best combination—vincristine and prednisone—produced a remission rate of over 90 percent, with relatively little toxicity.

For Tom, this was a truly spectacular achievement and the single most impressive event short of the actual achievement of cure in this disease. ''Imagine, a seven-year-old child comes to you with a diagnosis of acute lymphocytic leukemia, deathly ill with anemia, bleeding, fever, bone pain, enlarged lymph nodes, destined five years earlier to die within one to three months. Vincristine and prednisone therapy is started [as in Protocol VI, for example], and the patient is substantially better within a few days and by three weeks, the leukemia is gone and essentially all the aforementioned findings have reversed. At three weeks, the bone marrow aspiration is done and no leukemia cells are found. And this happened not just occasionally but in close to 100 percent of patients."

From this group of protocols came the key insight that using drugs with different modes of action (and thus different kinds of toxicities) allowed one to use full doses of each drug, rather than just a little of each. The effect was at least additive and perhaps synergistic. (Multidrug treatment of tuberculosis had beaten the problem of bacterial resistance in the same way.)

Yet patients were still dying of leukemia. They were not dying as quickly, and they might enjoy significantly longer periods of remission, but sooner or later they all relapsed. So the focus shifted to trying to prevent the relapse. Could they keep the remissions going by continuing to give chemotherapy during remission? "We did not know for certain why patients relapse. Was it due to persistent microscopic disease that became drug resistant? Was it due to reinduction of the leukemia process, or were other factors involved, such as sanctuaries that drugs could not reach? Moreover, even if the mechanism of relapse did involve persisting microscopic disease, one could argue that it might be better not to treat patients in complete remission since such treatment was toxic and, while it might prolong the duration of remissions, it might also result in selection of resistant leukemia cell lines and thus decrease the opportunity for a second remission. Yet Abe Goldin had just demonstrated that the cure of mouse leukemia was much more likely to be achieved against a microscopic, as compared to a large, tumor mass or burden, as it was called. If this were applicable to patients, then a cure might require treatment during remission."

Protocol IV set up a double-blind experiment to see whether a complete remission (established by prednisone treatment) could be prolonged by treatment with other drugs (or placebos) during remission. Neither the doctor or patient knew whether the patient was getting 6-MP or the placebo—except, that is, by the length of the remission. It turned out that the group treated with 6-MP had remissions lasting, on the average, ten months; the control group, only two months. This established the fact that an agent that was good at getting a remission started was also likely to be effective at quelling residual microscopic disease. "This was a landmark study. Since we had reached the ultimate goal in complete remission rate—that is, greater than 90 percent—further quantitative studies of remission induction would not make statistical sense. Our quantitative target thus became the duration of the remission. Clearly we were on the right track, but we had to do better."

The next step was to figure out whether dosage made a significant difference in the length of remissions. St. Jude's results in Protocol V made it clear that doubling the dose of a three-drug combination more than doubled the remission's duration. A surprising observation in Protocol VI was that the schedule of administration could also have a major effect; continuous daily doses were much less effective than a once-every-four-days schedule. Up to then, everyone had assumed that the schedule made no difference. But the study showed that the scheduling is critically important for certain drugs (for example, methotrexate and cytosine arabinoside [ara-c]) that attack cancer cells at specific stages in their growth and division. A current theory, based on test tube experiments by Doctors Robert Shimke and Joseph Bertino on methotrexate resistance in tumor cells, argues that continuous exposure of cells to the drug triggers gene amplification of the target enzyme, making the cells much more resistant to further exposure to the drug.

Protocol VIII was the famous VAMP program, using four drugs in combination. Tom's story of its beginning exemplifies the close professional relationship and friendship between himself and J.

"In early 1962, J and I were having one of our usual late afternoon discussions about the direction of our research. In going over our studies from the previous seven years, we noted that two agents were better than one; that two followed shortly by one was better than two only; and that two (vincristine, prednisone) followed in three weeks by two were better yet. In tuberculosis and some other infectious diseases, two agents were better than one but three were better than two. Finally, all the basic science arguments for combinations of two agents applied even more compellingly for more than two agents. In terms of intensification, the four active agents for acute lymphocytic leukemia included two which did not suppress normal bone marrow functions. This meant that the summation dose intensity, if you will, could be augmented. In reviewing this data, the lights suddenly turned on. Why not use all four agents at once as intensively as possible and as early in the treatment of the patient (that is, the first treatment) as possible? J was just as sure that it was his idea as I am that it was my idea. Actually, it was derivative of the successive studies which we had conducted—it was an idea whose time had come."

The VAMP program also demonstrated the interweaving of results from studies of one kind of cancer with work on another. Acute lymphocytic leukemia, Hodgkin's disease, and non-Hodgkin's lymphoma all responded to the same four drugs, and all three kinds of cancer were treated according to the same principles in VAMP (and later variations of it).

Of the seventeen patients treated with VAMP, three continued in long-term disease-free survival. That is, they were cured. The patients who did relapse did so at a median time of 150 days, consistent in the model with almost, but not total, leukemia eradication. Parenthetically, the Acute Leukemia Group B studies that included vincristine and prednisone for complete remission induction, followed by the combination of 6-MP and methotrexate, also produced a handful of long-term survivors and a long duration of unmaintained remission.

The MOPP program for Hodgkin's disease derived from this, using nitrogen mustard, oncovin or vincristine, prednisone, and procarbazine. It produced not only a high rate of complete remissions (70–80 percent) but a cure rate of 40 percent to 50 percent. The cure rate was also in the range of 40 percent for patients with non-Hodgkin's lymphoma.

"Why did we do so well in the lymphomas and relatively less well in acute lymphocytic leukemia? I believe it had to do with the pharmacologic sanctuary, that is, meningeal leukemia, something which has grown into a major problem as our systemic treatment has gotten progressively better and something which was not a problem in patients with Hodgkin's disease."

The comparison of the results on the three different cancers in Protocol VIII forced the Acute Leukemia Group to look carefully at the problem of leukemia cells in the brain (meningeal leukemia). The protocols so far had achieved a remarkable improvement in the prospects of anyone diagnosed with acute lymphocytic leukemia: over 90 percent of patients could be brought into complete remission, and the remission had been prolonged from two months on the average to more than a year. Now, when patients relapsed, it was because leukemia cells had migrated to the central nervous system (CNS), found "pharmacological sanctuary" inside the brain, and multiplied there. The antileukemia drugs, however, could not pass through the blood-brain barrier except in concentrations too low to affect the inexorable increase of cancer cells in the brain. Protocols IX and X developed methods for killing the leukemia cells in the brain by injecting drugs directly into the spinal fluid and, more important, for irradiating the head—work that was done by Dr. Donald Pinkel at St. Jude (see Chapter 12).

Complementing the clinical trials was preclinical research, primarily by Dr. Howard Skipper (see Chapter 10), on the L_{1210} mouse leukemia model, which provided a theoretical basis for interpreting the results of the protocols. The collaboration of Skipper and Tom Frei was a direct result of both the protocols and another program started by Gordon Zubrod; they were both members of the Acute Leukemia Task Force that Zubrod had founded in 1960 as a means of bringing together scientists and physicians who were working on therapeutic research in leukemia.

Skipper showed Tom that in the L_{1210} mouse leukemia model, the duration of a remission from the time treatment ended to the time of relapse was directly proportional to the number of leukemia cells left when treatment stopped. Tom immediately began looking at his clinical data with the model in mind.

These were the key clinically related discoveries, as Tom reflects on the cure of childhood leukemia. "That's the story! That's how curative treatment was developed for acute lymphocytic leukemia, but it is far from telling the whole story. The sequence of protocols really represents a scientific side of the achievement. Science can also be intensely personal and full of emotion, particularly when applied to the clinic. But there is also a much more intensely personal side of therapeutic research—the physician relationship with the patient. Patients who enter and agree to enter therapeutic research programs for cancer are indeed a select group. Almost without exception, they were very special—full of affection, curiosity, and most particularly, courage. This applied variably to the patients, depending upon their age, as well as to their parents."

It may sound cold and impersonal to talk about protocols, but to do so is a shorthand for describing therapeutic relationships with many patients. Although we may not foresee it, ultimately the work is all about caring for sick people, like Susan and Ernie.

"About the time I was appointed chief of the Leukemia Service, I had a patient by the name of Susan Jones, a seven-year-old girl recently diagnosed with acute lymphocytic leukemia, with whom I identified very strongly. She was a lovely youngster, and I got to know her almost as well as my own daughters. I was close to her parents, too—her father was a minister. When she came, she was at death's door, suffering from all the complexities of her disease. But on treatment with methotrexate, she entered and stayed in a complete remission for quite a long period of time. She then had a relapse, but we were able to get her into a second remission with ACTH, the corticosteroid drug we were using then.

"Susan then developed bleeding complications. She had fever, bone pain, anemia; she looked pale; she was bleeding from the eyes, nose, and mouth. Even her parents almost wrote her off. I stayed with her through a couple of nights, worried with her through the new platelet transfusions and the limited chemotherapy we had at the time. She got better, gradually at first; and then quite rapidly, a lot better. In fact, she went into a complete remission and went home.

"To be able to do this with a lovely child like that, whom you think of almost as your own, is truly an extraordinary experience. It has had a lot to do with my going into therapeutic research in cancer. Many doctors never have that kind of experience. But I did have the evidence that you could succeed. In the end you may fail—and when Susan relapsed yet again, it was devastating for me personally—but the fact that you could succeed in part meant that you could go all the way if you did it right. At least that was the attitude that I had, and that J and Jim Holland shared. It was born out of scientific insights, biochemical insights, insights from cancer chemotherapy and experimental models, but also the limited but deeply moving experiences one had with the Susan Joneses.

"The vast majority of the young people working on the Leukemia Service who had that kind of experience in fact dropped out of the field, didn't go into cancer research as a career. Those of us who did were in the minority, but we were a select minority: somehow we shared the feeling that we could succeed against the odds. There was a level of optimism and a positive approach among that group—Freireich, Holland, Zubrod, and myself—that I think everyone recognizes now in retrospect. Of the relatively few people in that age group who pioneered the field, virtually all shared that same positive attitude. And it's not surprising; because if you didn't have it, you couldn't stay in the field. There was no way that you could identify with Susan Jones and, having failed in the end, allow that failure to dominate your attitude."

Tom also identified strongly with Ernie Davis, an All-American football player from Syracuse. Over two or three Saturdays the young black athlete had played less and less well. At a clinic, blood counts showed him to be anemic. Eventually he was diagnosed as having acute myelogenous leukemia, and he was sent to the NCI for treatment around 1960. When he came, he was quite anemic, his platelet count was extremely low, and he was bleeding.

Tom had always been active in sports and he loved football, so he sympathized deeply with this bright enthusiastic young man who was never going to be able to play football again. At the time, Tom was testing methylbisguanylhydrazone (nicknamed methyl GAG), one of the first new drugs. It was a drug that had antileukemic activity, but was too toxic for general use. After four weeks of chemotherapy, Ernie had a complete remission: that is, no leukemic cells could be detected in the bone marrow tests. For four or five months he was actually able to go back to practice (though the doctors barred him from contact football).

Tom learned a great deal from Ernie, both about the natural history of leukemia and about courage. Ernie was unique among Tom's patients, because his livelihood depended on reaching and maintaining absolute peak physical performance. During his remission he did just about return to his accustomed peak level of capacity. As long as the leukemic cells could not be detected, his normal health was restored.

But Ernie relapsed, and no matter what the doctors tried, they could not achieve a second remission. Ernie died of complications from a nose-bleed that was almost impossible to stop.

"I remember vividly how terrifying nosebleeds were for leukemia patients and for me and the other young doctors who cared for them at NCI in those days before platelet transfusions. Patients like Ernie would start with a severe nosebleed. First, we'd try squeezing the patient's nose and put ice on it. When that did not stanch the bleeding, we'd pack gauze into the patient's nostrils. When that failed, we'd have to call in an ear, nose, throat specialist, who would go in through the mouth and pack the nasal passage from behind with gauze, which then had to be pulled forward into the nose. The idea was to apply pressure on the blood vessels from inside the nose. But the pack made patients miserably uncomfortable, and it rarely controlled the bleeding completely. As soon as the gauze was taken out, the bleeding would start again. All too often, devastating bacterial and fungal infections would invade first the nose, then the sinuses, and then move into the brain or the bloodstream. That is what happened to Ernie Davis. Over and over he had to be packed for nosebleeds; eventually he developed bleeding in the brain and died of brain hemorrhage and infection."

All through this ordeal, Ernie kept telling Tom to keep trying whatever he could; he was glad to be in a place where doctors were willing to try out new drugs and treatments. He was, for example, one of the first patients to receive a platelet transfusion. Although it did not help him because it was a case of too little too late, Ernie found it consoling to know that what Tom learned from his case might eventually help others.

Any doctor who works on a disease as critical and life-threatening as leukemia has to be driven by hope. Otherwise, the failures become overwhelming. Hope can always stand reinforcement, and Tom found that it worked both ways. "As a physician, there's a certain compatibility you have with your patients, or lack of compatibility, at the time—it's not written about very much, but it's there. If there is a lack of compatibility, you may do everything possible as a doctor, but you can't make that bridge of compatibility. Those tend to be the patients you don't remember. The patients you do remember are the ones who had courage, those who joined the battle for its own sake, and the ones like Susan Jones and Ernie Davis on whom you worked extra hard."

Ernie's case and many others like it underscored the necessity of finding better ways to care for patients while chemotherapeutic measures to bring them into (or back into) remission were tried. If the patient died of bleeding or infection before the drugs had time to work, you had helped neither the patient nor the progress of the drug research. So Tom feels particular pride at his share in pioneering the field of platelet and white blood cell transfusions. "All of that happened around 1962 and 1963, and I can vividly remember the excitement."

That excitement was strong at NCI, where Frei, Freireich, and their colleagues now felt quite secure about their work. They had by this time built up a critical mass of researchers there with interrelated and shared goals. They had administrators who understood those goals. Through the cooperative groups, they had close ties with investigators at other institutions and knew that they were all coming to similar conclusions about leukemia treatment. They had a staff of nurses committed to the research endeavor, and they had patients who had deliberately chosen to be "guinea pigs" in exchange for free treatment and—far more important—for hope.

But nay-sayers abounded in and out of NCI. There were plenty of young NCI fellows who, despite their presumed interest in research, could not see why their patients endured all the procedures and toxicity that the research protocol required. "You have to understand the setting: acute leukemia in children was a dreadful disease, and once the diagnosis was made, it was all over. Everyone who visited us, everybody we talked with, every textbook on the subject said that you cannot cure the disease, and you ought to give patients your best supportive care, keep them comfortable at home, and what have you. Very few people thought that an investment in the disease made any sense at all. People constantly advised me to go into other fields because they thought we weren't going to make any progress. They were trying to be helpful with their advice, but of course when you resisted it, they wondered about your sanity."

The beginning success didn't stop the hostility. In fact in some ways the hostility became worse at the point when it first appeared that some of the patients might be cured. When the results at NCI were so much better than those anywhere else, a lot of doctors didn't believe them and a lot, if not most, of the senior hematologists in the country didn't either. But the history of medicine is full of disbelievers who have turned out to be wrong.

"Indeed the realization that leukemia had been cured was very subtle and slow. It's very difficult to discuss the cures, because we tend to shortcut what actually happened. I seem to remember from high point to high point. But there wasn't any one point in time when we could say, 'OK, we're at a watershed, and now we are curing patients.' When national mortality statistics came along, we found out how many patients were dying of what diseases. Acute childhood leukemia is not so common: there are about 2,000 deaths a year in the United States, and death rate was 100 percent. Starting around 1965, there was a little bit of improvement, and fewer patients were dying of the disease than were contracting it. That was progressively improved, so that fifteen years later, in 1980, it was down to 50 percent. But there wasn't a single headline in a newspaper that said, 'Leukemia is cured as of December 30, 1965'—it didn't happen that way. True, in retrospect it seemed that fewer patients were dying, but no statistics were available to prove that impression. But there was a good deal of publicity between 1975 and 1980 as the news got out that the death rate of leukemia had been cut in half: there was no question that this represented progress. But that, in turn, incited not only hostility but a lot of doubt. I am not happy to have to say so, but at the same time it would be wrong to pretend it didn't exist."

The opposition expressed by the NCI blood bank director's flat dismissal of all treatment research on leukemia was symptomatic of skepticism echoed by other senior hematologists in the country. Every time Frei, Freireich, and their colleagues submitted a paper to *Blood* and other major journals in the field or gave a talk at the International Hematology Conference, the critics responded in force. Two prominent and influential hematologists, Dr. William Crosby and Dr. William Dameshek, wrote frequent editorials to the effect that there was no basis to thinking that leukemia was curable and that the investigators should let these patients alone. One widely quoted article said that acute leukemia was tougher than the patient and certainly tougher than the doctor, so there was no point in treating such patients. Such outspoken opposition to the NCI's work was bound to have an impact on doctors who found themselves treating leukemia patients.

"If you're a prestigious expert and you've been saying that something is one way for a long time and then a couple of young bucks come along and tell you it's the other way, that often creates hostility. I think it was late 1963 when Dr. Ken Endicott, then the director of NCI, asked me to make a presentation to the National Cancer Advisory Board about treatment strategies. This was an important group, so I talked about our VAMP program for leukemia and the MOPP program for Hodgkin's disease.

"I explained the experimental and theoretical bases for them, and why we thought these new programs might possibly be curative. I explained why we were justified in doing studies in patients involving multiple drugs and giving them supportive care to keep them alive while we were deliberately creating some degree of toxicity from our drugs, by using them to their maximum doses.

"There was a senior hematologist on the National Cancer Advisory Board by the name of Dr. Carl Moore, who happened to be a friend of my father's from St. Louis. I had always considered him a friend too. But my presentation struck him as being outrageous. He didn't deal in pediatric diseases like childhood leukemia, so he talked about Hodgkin's disease in adults. He said that if you have a patient who has widespread Hodgkin's disease, then it's best to tell that patient to go to Florida and enjoy life. If patients are having too many symptoms from their Hodgkin's disease, you treat them with a little x-ray or possibly a little nitrogen mustard, but give the smallest dose possible. Anything more aggressive than that is unethical, and giving four drugs at a time is unconscionable. He said this publicly before the National Cancer Advisory Board, before a lot of very distinguished advisory people, some of whom weren't even physicians. But when they heard the opinion of this very well respected man and then saw this young buck standing up in front of them, you can bet that my back was to the wall.

"Well, I never got mad. I told Dr. Moore that I understood his position, but I hoped he understood mine, and that what we were trying to do was something different. That was the very purpose of the National Cancer Institute. We weren't here to do the same things that he was doing at Washington University Hospital in St. Louis. If we were going to have a meaningful research program on leukemia and lymphoma, we *had* to do something different. After all, we had put together all the power of our collective intellect, motivation, and so on, and we also had the best experimentalists at the National Cancer Institute. After I finished, my colleague Dr. Lloyd Law got up, and he gave a talk very strongly in favor of my position. He was followed by Dr. Abe Goldin and other NCI colleagues who were also doing animal tumor research at NCI. That tended to balance things off a little, but nevertheless, the National Cancer Advisory Board voted to have an investigation of our program at NCI.

"That investigation wasn't too serious when it came, because by then we had a considerable amount of credibility among the senior staff of the institution. More important still, we had the data. But there was a meeting in the board room to investigate what we were doing. They weren't going to stop us from doing what we were doing, however. We were trying to save the lives of kids who would otherwise die for sure, and nobody was going to stop us from trying! Particularly when we'd had some, even though not the ultimate, success.

"So a formal censure did not happen, although that wasn't the end of it. Even then there were many good hematologists who would look at us strangely when we presented our data to them, and we knew from their reactions that we were losing them. They'd be thinking, 'Well, maybe he's not crazy, but there must be something wrong with the data. Somebody's telling him the wrong thing. Maybe if I talk to him he'll get over it.' That kind of thing was pretty common even with some of our mutual friends." Tom's comment is accurate.

The principles that were emerging from these lab and clinical studies not only profoundly influenced research on the basic biology of leukemia and the conduct of clinical trials; they also encouraged physicians studying other kinds of cancer to investigate whether the ideas held true for the treatment of those diseases as well. And when the leukemia research all came together, it made a big impact also on Hodgkin's disease and other lymphomas, and on breast and many other cancers. Tom published a very significant paper in 1966 entitled "Selected Considerations Regarding Chemotherapy as Adjuvant in Cancer Treatment." In it he develops the rationale that would guide chemotherapy to cure cancer after surgical removal of most of the cells.

With Hodgkin's disease, for example, the researchers put together the treatment program known as MOPP using four drugs, including three familiar from leukemia work: methotrexate, vincristine, and prednisone. Individually, each one of these drugs could produce complete remission in 10 to 20 percent of Hodgkin's disease patients; putting them all together seemed likely to kill 10^4 of the cancer cells, a much better result. It would not have been good enough for leukemia, where, as Skipper's and Frei's work had demonstrated, 10^{12} cells had to be destroyed. But in Hodgkin's disease, the number of actively dividing cells within the mass of the tumor was considerably lower than a trillion.

"Dr. Paul Carbone [who had shown that alkylating agents could produce remissions in Hodgkin's disease], Dr. Vincent DeVita [who had come as a clinical associate in 1963—and rose to be head of NCI years later], and I put our heads together and generated studies of combination chemotherapy that led to the cure of Hodgkin's disease.

"That was another very exciting period. It was very controversial because it was argued, as with the VAMP program, that we should look at all combinations of two and three drugs before proceeding to use all four agents together. In other words, it was argued that we should be more systematic. It would have taken some twenty to thirty studies and many years of testing to do this. Moreover, the MOPP program represented an inductive synthesis of the lessons we had learned from Hodgkin's disease and particularly from acute childhood leukemia. In those early studies of patients with Hodgkin's disease, we learned another lesson. What was especially compelling to me was the rapidity with which patients entered complete remission—that is, the rapidity of tumor destruction by multiple drugs—in contrast to single-agent treatment of Hodgkin's disease, where response was slow and occurred over many months and was usually at best partial. For MOPP-treated patients, response was fast, often dramatic, and at least half of the patients achieved complete remission within one or two months." As with leukemia, the intent was to use combination chemotherapy to produce complete remissions, to continue therapy even after visible evidence of cancer was gone, and only then to hope for and expect a cure.

One such patient is Les Willig, a businessman exactly the same age as Tom, and now more a friend than a patient. When he was first diagnosed with Hodgkin's disease in 1964, he went to seven or eight hematologists, all of whom told him essentially to go to Florida and make the best of it— very common advice at the time. Les wasn't willing to take that advice. He thought it was outrageous for these doctors to tell him they couldn't treat him. He finally hit on Howard Skipper, although Howard isn't a physician. But Howard sent him to Tom, because he was doing some of the first experiments on Hodgkin's disease. When Les first came, Tom treated him with curative intent, though they surely didn't know he was going to be cured. But he was.

"Every one of those patients who got caught in our net of enthusiasm and hope was swimming upstream because they, like Willig, had been told by other doctors that no one could do anything for them. So patients like Les Willig had real courage. They and their families weren't going to take no for an answer. The kids who went through had the hope that, if they took the intensive treatment, whether or not they had toxic side effects, they might have a chance to be the lucky ones. But the early patients all died. Subsequently people benefited, thanks to these pioneer patients. They were the laboratory that allowed that to be done."

From time to time when Tom gives an important presentation about Hodgkin's disease to medical students or young doctors, Les Willig will come all the way from Evansville, Indiana, to stand up as one of the first patients who had widespread disease and had failed extensive radiation and other chemotherapy who was cured of Hodgkin's disease. He will talk frankly about the frustrations of being told that nothing could be done to help him. And he is equally frank about the misery that patients are willing to go through to be cured. In 1980, when Tom first presented this case to a group, at grand rounds at Harvard's Peter Bent Brigham Hospital, Les was sitting in the first row, listening as Tom explained about the first use of combination therapy for the disease. The doctors asked Tom all kinds of questions about the side effects of the treatment, and also asked Les how he tolerated the treatments. Les looked at Dr. Frei and said: "I never told you I had so much nausea and vomiting, because I was afraid you wouldn't give me the next course of treatment. But, after you'd treat me, I'd go home and vomit for a week." Said Tom, "There was nothing, nothing that was going to stop him from getting that treatment. He would have walked through a wall."

In writing a book about the conquest of childhood leukemia, it is very tempting to describe the experiments that worked and omit the 95 percent that did not. At least some of the failures were just as logical and well conceived as those that won victories.

When I was a clinical associate on the Leukemia Service in the 1950s, Tom and J were trying something that seemed crazy to us: they were using a pig extract as an experimental treatment of leukemia. It was an awful project for all concerned, and we hated being part of its implementation. Yet it illustrated the desperation of the scientists to try virtually anything that had a chance for success and the desperation of the patients and parents to try it out. We had to prepare an extract of raw pig, make it into a liquid like a milkshake, and feed it to patients three times a day. It smelled awful, it tasted awful, and the children often vomited after a dose. What was the idea behind that? Tom finds it difficult to talk about, even thirty-five or more years later.

"Well, it's a little embarrassing, and I suppose both J and I are responsible for it. We never published it, but I can remember doing the first pigs. It truly was a crazy experiment, you're right about that, but at the time it didn't seem all that crazy. People outside of our field wouldn't know that in the medical literature of the 1920s physicians thought that pernicious anemia was a type of malignancy. Now, of course, we know that it was due to a deficiency of vitamin B_{12} and we can cure it, but one didn't know that then. When you looked at the bone marrow of patients with pernicious anemia, you saw these big, juicy, terrible-looking, early red cells filling up the marrow, getting into the spleen and lymph nodes, and then all of the patients with pernicious anemia died. With the information that was available at that time, the clinical picture resembled a malignancy that was just as malicious as, let's say, leukemia. Doctors couldn't go beyond that point until they discovered vitamin B_{12} and then they found that, when you gave that to patients with pernicious anemia, bam, they were cured. Of course it wasn't leukemia at all, only a strange vitamin deficiency effect. Well, we were thinking that possibly there might be a similar problem in the development of the white cells as opposed to the red cells that primarily are involved in pernicious anemia. Maybe we just needed to find the right vitamin that allowed those cells to mature and that the patients were lacking a key factor. If so, how do you find that factor?

"We didn't have any leads, of course, but we speculated that there was a vitamin that normal people without leukemia had and people with leukemia lacked. So we went to the laboratories and looked at strains of mice that genetically were predisposed to having a high incidence of leukemia and compared them with those that had a very low incidence of leukemia. We thought maybe there was something of that vitamin in the low leukemia strain, and so we killed the low leukemia strain mice and ground them up and fed them to the high leukemia strain. I know it sounds crazy as I am explaining it now. That experiment didn't work, but there are a lot of problems with doing experiments on inbred strains of mice anyway.

"Of course we couldn't cannibalize people, so we looked for a species considered to be closely related to man and for this purpose we chose pigs. The next thing we thought about was what part of the pig should we take—the liver, the spleen, or what have you? We really weren't sure what to do, and we didn't want to take a chance that we would arbitrarily select the wrong part of the pig, because the vitamin might be in the skin or might be in the central nervous system or any organ. So we decided that the only way to do this properly was to take the whole pig after the intestines had been removed.

"We went out to an experimental farm in Beltsville, Maryland, where animals were sacrificed, ground up, and prepared in a colloid mill. We used immature pigs, thinking that if there was a vitamin, surely the immature pigs would have the most of it. When pigs were processed through this colloid mill, we ended up with a product that looked like milkshakes. We couldn't heat or boil this material for fear of inactivating the protective factor. We kept pig 'milkshakes' in the refrigerator and freezer, and, as a matter of fact, that's what some people called them when they saw them sitting there in the freezer.

"I remember Laura, who had acute adult lymphocytic leukemia. She was so motivated and so nice; we were very close and I loved her dearly.

So I told her that I thought this was something that we ought to try after we had tried all of our other drugs. I didn't tell her the exact truth, I couldn't bring myself to do that, but I told her what the theory was and so forth. She swallowed a stomach tube and we fed her the pig extract by pouring it through that tube. Of course the content of fat in this stuff was so high that it just satiated her and caused her some nausea, when she wasn't feeling too well anyhow. But she was motivated, so she did this every day and it was the way she got her calories—from raw pig extract. We hoped that this nutritious stuff also contained an antileukemia factor, something that would do for leukemia what vitamin B_{12} did for pernicious anemia. Every day I would go down to the laboratory and look at her blood in the hopes that there would be some evidence of improvement, but there wasn't one shred of improvement. Then we worried that maybe we had done the wrong thing, that maybe the vitamin was somehow quite unstable and so we should have treated the tissues differently or we should have concentrated it or perhaps we should have worked with particular organs—and we thought about going through the whole business again. We finally gave it up as a bad go. We certainly didn't only do successful experiments and if there was ever any doubt, that experiment proved that point very well."

Fortunately, better days lay ahead. For Tom, the capstone to those years of many setbacks and slow incremental progress came in 1983, when he and J were awarded the General Motors Kettering Prize. At a press conference, a woman stepped over to Tom and said: "Dr. Frei, do you know who I am?" He looked at her and said, "No, ma'am, I'm sorry I don't." She told him her name and Tom said politely, "That's interesting." But then she added her maiden name. At that moment, he knew who she was: the second patient to be treated with the VAMP program back in 1961. She had been a terribly sick seven-year-old then. Now she was about thirty years old, with three children, as healthy and happy as could be. They hugged and hung on to each other for a long time. "Seeing her then, there was no question in my mind or in her mind. For her and for us, it had been a great success. And that was much more important to me than winning a prize."

The Blood
Cell Separator

I feel a special affection for the blood cell separator, the complex machine whose development caused so much grief to J Freireich, Tom Frei, George Judson, NCI, and IBM. IBM had decided that it would not be profitable for them to market the instrument. Subsequently, the technical plans, which were in the public domain and thus available to anyone, were picked up by Aminco, who thereby obtained all of the complex and expensive biomedical engineering free of charge, at least, to them.

The very first commercially produced separator (built by Aminco after IBM decided to drop the project) came to my laboratory at Duke University. My blood was the first to be separated as we tried out the new instrument. And I nervously witnessed the machine's first use on a leukemia patient.

At Duke, I was trying to find out how chemotherapy drugs actually kill human leukemia cells and how to predict which drug might be most effective for any given patient. We knew that different patients responded to different drugs, so we thought that it would be helpful to test each person's leukemia cells against a variety of drugs and then decide which drugs to use for that individual. To get enough cells, I used to remove 50 milliliters of blood, one-tenth of a pint, from a patient, add a fibrinogen solution to the syringe to settle out the red blood cells, and then push out the top layer of leukemic cells and plasma. The leukemic cells would be divided among many sterile flasks and incubated together with various radioactive nutrients and drugs for one or more days.

To conduct certain types of experiments, we knew that we needed much larger quantities of leukemia cells than we could safely get from patients by the method available. Thus, in 1970 I felt fortunate to be awarded a research grant to purchase the first blood cell separator to come off the production

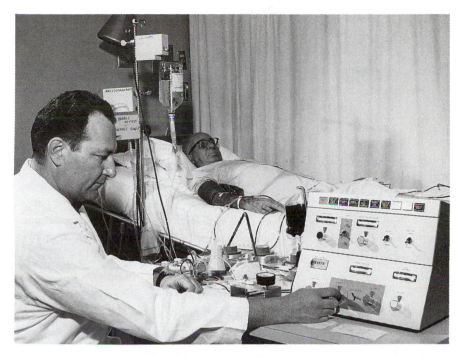

3. J Freireich at the controls of the first run with a patient on the IBM 2990 Blood Cell Separator in 1967. The instrument had been in clinical trials earlier at the National Cancer Institute. *(Courtesy of University of Texas, M. D. Anderson Hospital and Tumor Institute, Houston, Texas.)*

line. This instrument would enable us to remove billions of leukemia cells during a four-hour sitting while returning the red cells and plasma to the patient. It was a painless procedure and one that would also help the patient.

Despite all the testing the manufacturer does on its prototypes, it is still very anxiety provoking to put a new medical instrument into use. If something goes wrong, you can't just shut it off like a television set and call in someone to repair it—you are faced with a real patient, whose life is literally on the line, who is depending on its reliability. Our research nurses, Evelyn Morgan and Anna Vaughn, and my junior medical colleague, Dr. Donald S. Miller, had witnessed a demonstration at the National Cancer Institute; and when our new blood cell separator arrived at Duke, the chief Aminco technician came to test the components and help us with some practice runs. We tried it first on anesthetized dogs, and all went smoothly; then we planned to try it out on normal human volunteers.

Our clinical protocol carefully described the steps that we would follow. Two large-bore needles were attached to plastic catheters. One needle went into a vein of the left forearm of the person, the other in a right arm vein. Blood flowed out from one arm vein and into the machine, where the centrifuge separated it into its three chief components: plasma, red blood cells, and white blood cells (with platelets). On the far side of the separator, the two columns of red cells and plasma flowed back into a single tube and gently pumped back into a large vein in the other arm while the leukemia (or normal white) cells were removed by collecting them into a sterile blood bag.

The principle was really quite simple. Once the catheters were in place, our nurses and the technician took over the entire procedure, and the patient was free to watch television, talk, and eat. The only things a patient couldn't do were to get up to go to the bathroom or scratch an itch—two limitations that almost immediately evoked a need! The whole process of this early cell separator worked rather like a kidney dialysis machine, but it was designed to remove leukemic cells (or normal cells) rather than excretory wastes as in dialysis. Everyone who was hooked up to the separator—whether a volunteer or a patient—was first told about the procedure, warned of its possible side effects, given an opportunity to ask questions and reflect, and then asked to sign a consent form indicating a willingness to participate in the experiment.

Our staff volunteered first for the trial runs of the system. Because I had big juicy arm veins that were easy to stick, plus a major interest in using this technology, I was the first experimental subject. The needles and catheters were positioned in my veins and secured to the outer surface of my skin with tape. Blood flowed quickly from my right forearm into the centrifuge bowl. The brilliant engineering trick had been to design a closed system that would permit a continuous flow of blood in and out of a rapidly spinning centrifuge bowl. If it weren't totally airtight, we'd be splattering my blood all over the room. ACD solution, a preservative used in blood banking, was added to the blood to keep it from clotting in the tubes. A salt solution was initially pumped into my left forearm to replace the temporary loss of blood, a kind of "priming of the pump." Downstream from the bowl, soon after the start of the centrifugation, my separated red blood cells and plasma were combined into a single tube and returned to me. The normal white blood cells were separated out, to be examined later. The loss of these cells was not a problem: I had plenty of reserves in the bone marrow, and they rapidly replenished the blood.

All was going well with the initial run, and there were relieved smiles all around. Visiting staff, making lighthearted remarks about the doctor getting a taste of his own medicine, paraded in and out of the room to examine the remarkable new instrument that fractionated blood into its component parts while it flowed continuously. It was strange to see the tubes coming out of the machine with clear yellow plasma in one, deep red liquid in another, and a syrupy mixture of cells in the third. As my mind wandered, it conjured up the image of a beam of light separated into all of its rainbow-colored parts by a glass prism—only our new instrument could put all or some of the parts back together, just as we wished.

It seemed to be chilly in the room, and I asked for a blanket. Then my heart rate began to speed up, and I felt hot, cold, sweaty, and uncomfortable. Anna and Evelyn checked me over, measured my temperature, and it was all I could do to keep from biting the thermometer in half as I began shaking with chills. Dr. Miller checked me over, and we considered the possibility that one of the sterile plastic tubes or the sterile centrifuge bowl was not sterile after all, or that there was some contaminant that was causing an allergic or fever response. A blood culture test was drawn to search for bacterial contamination, but we knew that the results would not be available until long after the four-hour procedure was completed and that therefore it was of no help in our immediate dilemma—though it would help us sort out our future strategy. We stayed with the run for a while longer until it was clear that my reaction would not subside spontaneously; then we stopped the centrifuge and its pumps, pulled out the catheters, and put pressure over the site of the needle sticks. I was still shaking when we quit, but this stopped within fifteen minutes after I was disconnected from the machine. The blood fractionation had gone well, yet something was seriously wrong. I had no aftereffects, but obviously we were not ready to do this to sick patients.

It took us weeks of checking to find the problem. We changed the types of catheters, altered the method of sterilizing the bowl, used different intravenous solutions, and made other changes too numerous to mention. It turned out that the problem was not bacterial contamination but apparently came from a trace of metallic material, possibly aluminum, that was being washed off from the inside of the centrifuge bowl. This substance was never fully identified, but it caused chills and fever—until we were finally able to remove it completely during the process of repeatedly washing and steriliz-ing the bowl. Thereafter we had no more trouble until we changed to a new bowl some months later. This time we fixed it quickly, and what we learned at Duke ultimately led to the development of better bowl materials and the resolution of this problem for all other hospitals, as they later began to install their own instruments. We ran the cell separator procedure on other staff members and then on paid student and staff volunteers, until we were ready to go with a real leukemia patient.

The emergency call came in late on a hot Friday afternoon. A general practitioner from a town in eastern North Carolina urgently wanted to speak to a blood specialist—anyone who was available. One of my colleagues took the call. The physician had a patient, a twenty-year-old hairdresser, who had come to see him with a story of feeling faint for a day or two and having experienced a sudden partial loss of vision in her right eye. Upon examination, he found a few bruises on her skin, hemorrhages in both eyes, severe anemia, and a white blood cell count that was "too high to measure."

When Betty arrived at Duke at around 8 P.M., she looked like a frightened deer, ready to bolt, but afraid to make a sound. The intern, the resident, and attending doctors had many questions. Her mother answered most of them for her. Betty looked like a teenager, with her hair in a ponytail and wearing a colorful print dress. Her pulse was rapid, her blood pressure low, and her breathing shallow and rapid as she panted for air. Her leukemic cells were using up so much of the blood oxygen that her tissues were hungry for oxygen. She had severe anemia. Tiny hemorrhages as well as large blotches covered her skin, particularly on her arms and legs; hemorrhages covered the macular portion of the right eye, which accounted for her partial loss of vision.

Her spleen and liver were very large and tender. She cried out with pain when I applied mild finger pressure over the bones of her sternum and pelvis, an indication that the bone marrow was expanding rapidly. Even without looking at a blood film, the diagnosis of leukemia was quite obvious. And her white cell count was 294,000 cells per cubic milliliter of blood— about thirtyfold higher than normal. Even more important was the fact that, examined under the microscope, the large immature white blood cells were typical of those seen in acute leukemia. Indeed, it was difficult to find any normal white cells among the leukemic ones. During the time we were examining her, making our decisions, and assembling our blood cell separator team, she became progressively more lethargic and difficult to rouse.

We urgently had to reduce the number of leukemic cells, or risk a fatal hemorrhage in the brain—an all too common and rapid complication of a very high leukemic cell count. We called the cell separator team together to explain the problem to them, and the technician, two nurses, and Dr. Miller assumed their stations. We began as soon as Betty's mother and boyfriend had also been fully informed and had urged Betty to participate in the cell separator program: they all agreed. Indeed, there was virtually no other choice, and they were fortunate to be at the one hospital that had this new technology. The next twenty-four to forty-eight hours were critical; her long-term survival hinged on our ability to pull her through the present emergency. We could not treat her leukemia until the sheer number of white cells had been brought down. As far as we were concerned, there would never be a more convenient time to put the blood cell separator into use, even though we all felt trepidation about making its first trial on someone so desperately ill.

The procedure itself went well. The many hours of practice paid off in flawless teamwork. The huge numbers of white cells that came from the blood cell separator resembled cream as they flowed out of the machine, through the tube and into separate blood bags that were quickly chilled on ice and taken to the laboratory for study.

Immediately following this four-hour leukopheresis procedure, as it's called, Betty's white count had dropped to 50,000 and she was out of imminent danger. Betty felt good and far more mentally alert when it was over; I doubt she realized how relieved we all were that the procedure had gone so well. Betty went back to her hospital room, had a good snack, and fell asleep. Then our laboratory team, the basic scientists, took over and worked all night to prepare fresh enzymes from her leukemic cells that would be used for further research studies.

We immediately started chemotherapy by intravenous infusion, but since chemotherapy would take days to have an effect, we had to repeat the cell separator procedure again on Monday. By then her count had risen to 175,000, but the separator brought it down to 37,000; thereafter, it did not go back up again. As the drugs took effect, the white count leveled off, then plummeted, as the leukemia cells in the blood and bone marrow were killed off.

For the next three weeks, the staff dealt with the complication of very low red and white blood counts. We had to transfuse enough red blood cells to maintain normal tissue oxygen levels. Betty needed dozens of platelet transfusions, obtained from the Red Cross, to keep her from bleeding spontaneously. We also used powerful antibiotics to treat serious infections in her bloodstream and lungs until we reached the point when her normal white blood cells began to reappear. A bone marrow test was repeated and revealed that about 70 percent of her cells were now normal, but the remaining 30 percent were still leukemic.

Betty was treated again with chemotherapy and developed ulcers on her lips and in her mouth and throat. It was painful for her to eat, drink, or even swallow her saliva, and her voice became hoarse and raspy. She was particularly dismayed when her hair came out in clumps as her mother brushed it. The infections reappeared, she developed a painful abscess near her rectum, and she again required continuous intravenous fluids, antibiotics, and other medications. She felt too ill and embarrassed to have visitors other than her boyfriend and her mother. Everyone who entered the room had to wear a gown and mask to minimize the risk of bringing in other potentially infectious organisms. Such isolation from normal human contact creates a strange world, and for good reasons she became depressed. The nurses and Louise Bost and her Recreation Therapy staff worked with her. Betty found them much less threatening than the doctors and managed to while away some pleasant hours talking with her new friends.

Gradually, the vision in her right eye returned to normal, which she rightly took as a positive sign of recovery. When her normal white cells rose above the danger line, the gowns and masks came off and the smiles not only returned, but could be seen! Betty began to walk about the ward, watch television, and sew in the patient lounge, and she was glad to see her own friends when they came to visit. She wore a turban or other head covering to hide her patchy hair, and she dressed in casual clothes, rather than hospital pajamas, for most of the day. Soon she was well enough to have all the medicines discontinued, except for those that could be taken orally or given to her every three weeks as an outpatient, and Betty was discharged.

She left the hospital in a wheelchair, as is the custom, although she was strong enough to walk. Tears were shed as she said good-bye and embraced several of the nurses with whom she had become quite close. The doctors, particularly the resident and fellows, were very proud. Thereafter her bone marrow rapidly regained its normal cells, and her liver and spleen shrank to normal size. Her hair eventually grew back, maybe a little curlier than before chemotherapy. She looked like her former self, but very much more poised. She went back to work and within a few months she married her high school sweetheart, though both knew that she was not cured of her leukemia. One or two of the staff attended the wedding, a very special occasion for a brave young couple.

Our first blood cell separator experience had clearly been a success. We were to use that instrument and others thousands of times in the years to follow, often with equally dramatic effect, in leukemia, certain other blood, and even neurologic disorders.

PART IV

The
Periphery

CHAPTER 10

Howard Earle Skipper, Ph.D.

Nature wasn't trained as we were.
—Howard Skipper

Howard Skipper, Ph.D., calls himself a "mouse doctor" and confesses to puzzlement at being included here among the "real doctors" he so admires. As he looks back on his life as a biochemist in cancer research, he frets that "it has always seemed to take me inordinately long to recognize principles which in retrospect were really quite simple." His colleagues in cancer research, though, would laugh at these demurrals. They know that his work on leukemia in mice provided an essential model for treating human patients. They also know that Howard's "inordinately slow" insights were critical to the remarkably quick development of effective chemotherapy for leukemia in the mid- to late 1960s. Their respect for him and for the institution he created, the Southern Research Institute, is enormous.

Howard Skipper's career in biomedical science could not have been predicted from his family background or his early interests. His ancestors had settled in Florida well before the state was admitted to the Union. His parents were schoolteachers; then his father went into banking, real estate, and cattle ranching in Sebring, a little boom town in the center of the state. His brothers continued in the cattle-ranching tradition, but it held little appeal to Howard: "I spent so much time on a farm in my youth that, if I never see another cow, it'll be too soon."

During the Depression, the boom in Sebring collapsed, the family fell on hard times, and Howard was glad of a football scholarship to the University of Florida at Gainesville. He appreciated the room, board, and tuition, but not the two or three hours a day of "head knocking." As a second-string center on a mediocre team, "I never got to carry the ball unless I was intercepting a pass while backing up the line—a rare event." To earn pocket money, Howard tutored his fellow football players in remedial English and math, an experience that dissuaded him from going into teaching.

Howard was no more impressed with the faculty than with the football team. "The University of Florida wasn't too good a school at that time. The professors were sort of lazy." He had planned to become a lawyer, but his courses in economics, accounting, and business administration bored him. Only the chemistry professor—whose class he took by chance—impressed him, and he went on to take more courses in the subject.

Although he changed his mind about majors several times, he ultimately decided to go on to graduate school to study chemistry, biochemistry, nutrition, and biology. "The anatomy courses were rather dull, but I still remember such 'useful' information as the location of the pre- and post-zygapophyses. I rushed through graduate school in three years, working summers, because World War II seemed imminent. My outstanding achievement in graduate school undoubtedly was meeting, courting, and marrying a beautiful law student whose name became Margaret Skipper. (In 1940 the student body of the University of Florida comprised about 3,200 males and about 15–20 females, so this observation may be classified as bragging.)"

Two weeks after Howard received his doctorate, the letter from the President of the United States came, inviting him to join the army as a second lieutenant. This was in June 1941, almost six months before Pearl Harbor. His training in chemistry and biology brought an assignment to the Medical Research Division of the Chemical Warfare Service at Edgewood Arsenal in Maryland.

The only professional staff worthy of the name when Lt. Skipper arrived at Edgewood was an organic chemist, Dr. Seymour Silver. Howard credits Dr. Silver with teaching him more about chemistry in two years than all his professors had taught him. It was Silver who introduced him to the theories of ionization of the Swedish Nobel laureate (1903) Svante August Arrhenius, concerning the kinetics that describes cell killing in terms of the reaction rate between chemicals and the vital targets in the cells—fundamental work that had been published in 1910, but not taught at Florida. Silver also told Howard about the decades-old debate raging between chemists and biologists over the interpretation of data on bacteria exposed to various chemicals in the test tube; the significance of the precise shapes of those exponential curves relating dose to number of cells killed would continue to preoccupy Howard when he moved into cancer research.

At Edgewood Arsenal, Skipper's task was to synthesize derivatives of mustard gas, test their toxicity, and devise ways to protect against them. He still bears scars on his arms from deliberately trying out their irritating effects on himself.

In 1943 the Army sent Howard to Australia's Barrier Reef to join a British-Australian-American team that was studying the biological effects of chemical warfare agents and the ability of clothing, masks, and gloves to protect soldiers from poison gases. Howard and his team would set up chemical traps in bottles as sampling stations on the various islands of the region. Then "our people" would bomb the deserted islands with mustard gas. Two or three days later, Howard and his team, dressed in protective gear, would collect the sampling bottles and analyze how much mustard gas vapor had been trapped in the bottles.

"We were seriously trying to see how effective chemical warfare would be. For example, prior to the invasion of the island of Tarawa, the air force had bombed the island very extensively, and we still had about 4,500 casualties. Our High Command was well aware that there were many more islands ahead on the way to Japan. There was no question that the Japanese defending these islands were going to die, since they would not surrender. The question that was asked was whether American casualties could be prevented by the use of gas. We could have done that, but General MacArthur didn't wish to use poison gas, and consequently it was never used as a weapon. I'm very glad, because I think it's a terrible weapon, but we did extensive testing with it nonetheless. The Japanese didn't have good protective clothing, although they did have gas masks.

"We learned a lot in the two years I was there about the behavior of mustard gas in the atmosphere, and especially about the very high concentrations of gas that could be held close to the ground by jungle foliage or by temperature inversions. I learned firsthand about an important pharmacologic principle: the toxicity of some drugs is the product of the drug's concentration in the tissues it affects multiplied by the length of exposure time [toxicity = concentration $\times$ time, or $C \times T$]."

What this means is that the human body (and other biological systems) can tolerate high doses of certain toxic drugs if the period of exposure is very brief; but, if the same dose is given over a long period of time—or even a much lower dose given over a very long time—it can be fatal. Even though the antimetabolite drugs that became key in leukemia chemotherapy did not follow this rule, Howard's experience at looking at the interplay of toxicity, dose, and exposure proved invaluable in his later leukemia research. Clearly the intent of mustard gas in biological warfare is to maximize the toxicity against vital normal cells, whereas in cancer chemotherapy the goal is to optimize the killing of cancer cells according to their growth or other unique characteristics, minimizing toxicity as much as possible. The true impact of $C \times T$ depends upon whether the toxic agent irreversibly binds to its cellular target, as does mustard gas, or whether it only competes with normal metabolites during the time when the cell is dividing.

For Howard, like many other scientists, the Chemical Warfare Service was the training ground for his later efforts to save lives from cancer. Howard, for example, first paid attention to bone marrow cells because mustard agents strikingly inhibited the normal development of those cells. He tried very hard to find a way to reverse the inhibitory effects, but neither he nor anyone else found an effective antidote. That work was followed up at Edgewood Arsenal by two pharmacologists, Alfred Gilman and Fred Phillips, who turned the problem on its head: if the mustard agents inhibited normal cell growth, what would they do to cancerous cells? Just before the war's end, Gilman and Phillips, along with other colleagues, showed that nitrogen mustard could bring about temporary remissions in patients with lymphoma—quite possibly the first time any drug had worked at all on any kind of cancer. Even though the mustard-based drugs did not prove very useful against the cancerous bone marrow cells of leukemia, their demonstration that something could be done against another blood-cell-derived and often widespread cancer like lymphoma gave chemotherapy research on leukemia an enormous psychological boost.

For the history of leukemia research, the friendships formed in the Chemical Warfare Service that continued after the war may have been as important as the lines of scientific thinking that started there. The Skippers' neighbor at Edgewood Arsenal, Dr. David Karnofsky, for example, went on to work with Joe Burchenal at Memorial Sloan-Kettering and became a link between Joe and Howard. Dr. C. P. Rhoads, the new chief of the research program in the Chemical Warfare Service and Karnofsky and Burchenal's future boss at Memorial Sloan-Kettering, became good friends with Howard during the six months they overlapped at Edgewood before Howard left for Australia. After the war, Rhoads tried to recruit Howard to join the Memorial Sloan-Kettering team, but Howard decided that New York was not for him: he wanted to do research, but in the South. When an Alabama physician, Dr. Wilbur Lazier, and a businessman, Ben May, approached Skipper about starting a new free-standing research institute in Birmingham, Rhoads generously introduced Howard to Alfred P. Sloan and Charles Kettering, the philanthropists who supported his own program. Their donations gave the Southern Research Institute a sound financial footing—and gave Howard a home for the rest of his career. He was on particularly good terms with "Boss" Kettering, the General Motors engineer who had made a fortune by inventing the self-starter for cars. Kettering was so interested in the scientific work at the fledgling institute that he would often fly down from his home in Dayton to find out what was new, and Howard would sometimes fly back with him to continue their conversation.

From Rhoads, Skipper also learned the importance of cultivating links between scientists like himself who did basic research and those who applied the research to humans in clinical settings. The collaboration between Memorial Sloan-Kettering and Southern Research Institute continued until Rhoads's death in 1959. Then it shifted to the new center of leukemia research, Dr. Gordon Zubrod's group at the National Cancer Institute.

"I had an excellent working relationship with Gordon's Acute Leukemia Task Force [1962–1968] and with his later ad hoc Chemotherapy Advisory Group [1969–1974]. The first group was made up of physicians [Frei, Freireich, Holland], pharmacologists, chemists, and other scientists. We started with eight or ten people, but gradually everyone else wanted to come. That diluted the value of the meetings, and they petered out. Later Gordon said he'd like to try to set it up again, but not to tell everyone! Frei and Freireich were then in Houston, Zubrod and the NCI people were in Bethesda, and Frank Schabel and I were in Birmingham, so Atlanta was convenient for all of us. We'd meet in an Atlanta motel for a day and a half. Certain people would bring in their data—both clinical and laboratory data—and we'd criticize it. The discussions got pretty spirited: I remember losing my temper with one person (guess who!) and asking him to go outside and conduct his argument out there if he couldn't behave himself. But pretty soon we began talking the same language, clinicians and basic scientists alike."

That was an accomplishment in itself. It is hard for basic scientists and clinical scientists to work together successfully. Their training is different, the literature they read is different, and often their temperaments and levels of patience are different. The clinical scientists often feel like lay people when it comes to appreciating the lab techniques, data, and methodology of the experimentalist. For the experimentalists, the difficulty comes in not understanding the medical realities, the ways the animal model or tissue culture system they are studying in the lab differs from what is going on in patients—indeed, the scientific and practical difficulty of conducting clinical research. But, as Howard once emphasized in a major address to the American Association for Cancer Research, "Nature wasn't trained as we were." There is no telling where discoveries are going to originate, or how a conversation between two people working in different areas, with different points of view, can bring about an advance that neither could have made alone.

Howard Skipper's important contributions to the interdisciplinary discussions on leukemia came with the work he and his colleague Frank Schabel did on the response of cancer cells to drugs, using a particular strain of leukemia, L_{1210}, in mice. "The point of our discovery was that a given dose of a drug will kill the same *percentage* of cancer cells with which it comes in contact, not the same *number* of cells. Thus, if a given drug has the capacity of killing 99.99 percent of the cells, it will do so regardless of whether there were one million or one billion cells to begin with. Well, that one-hundredth of one percent of cells that are not killed will be left behind to grow back another tumor—unless, of course, more drug, or a different drug, is added before the tumor has regenerated itself. This naturally led to the realization that we had to find schedules of drugs to kill cells faster than they were able to grow back. Only in that way could we ever hope to get the number of leukemic cells to zero, and thereby cure the animal."

First, Skipper and Schabel had to prove that a single leukemic cell could grow out so many daughter cells that they would eventually kill the animal. "From a leukemic mouse, take a single drop of blood—which may contain 100,000 leukemic cells—and with the aid of a fancy piece of equipment called a micromanipulator, pick out a single leukemia cell and carefully inject it into a healthy mouse. If you do that, two things will happen.

"The first is that the single leukemia cell, if it is a living, functional cell, will divide and form two leukemia cells; and these two will divide to form four; and then the four will become eight; and the eight, sixteen; the sixteen, thirty-two, and so on. until the number reaches about one billion. At that point, there are leukemia cells present in essentially every tissue and organ of the body, and the animal dies.

"The second is that it will have taken about fifteen days for that single leukemia cell and its progeny to proliferate up to one billion, which is the lethal number of a mouse. [In people, the lethal number of leukemia cells is closer to one trillion.] That tells us, in the case of the mouse, that our single leukemia cell and its progeny were doubling in number on the average of every half-day, or quadrupling in number every day [see table]."

Leukemia Cell Growth in Mice

Day	Number of leukemia cells
0	1
1	$4 = 2^2$
2	$16 = 2^3$
3	64
4	256
5	1,024
6	4,096
7	16,384
8	65,536
9	262,144
10	1,048,576
11	4,194,304
12	16,777,216
13	67,108,864
14	268,435,456
15 (death)	1,073,741,824 $= 2^{30}$
	($2^{30} =$ ca. $10^9 =$ ca. 1 gram of leukemia cells)

NOTE: This exponential, or logarithmic, pattern of rapidly expanding cell growth is characteristic of leukemia and of tumors in their early stages in animals and humans. Most tumor cells stop dividing quite so rapidly after the tumor reaches a certain size, so tumors do not grow or reach the lethal point as quickly.

Once Skipper and Schabel knew that the leukemic cells increased exponentially and at what rate, they could try all sorts of variations and interpret the results against the standard they had established. For example, if treated mice survived for twenty days rather than fifteen, then it was possible to calculate how many cells the treatment must have killed. Or, if the cancer was a tumor rather than leukemia, they tried removing the main mass surgically, and then used the drugs to kill the rest.

''The inescapable implication of these experiments is that in order to cure this mouse leukemia, we must kill every living leukemia cell in the mouse no matter where it is in the body, or else it will grow back to kill the mouse when it divides up to the magic number of about one billion. If there were one million cells in the animal at the time that we started treatment, and if our treatment killed 999,999—leaving a single cell alive— we would have failed, because that one malignant cell would give rise to one billion about fifteen days later. That's a stark reality. Another reality is that, if we are going to kill every last leukemia cell, we must choose drugs that will get into every organ and tissue and once there, will selectively kill leukemia cells. Furthermore, they must kill the leukemia cells faster than they're being replaced, and do so for a long enough period of time to reduce the number of cells to zero *and* without ever overdosing the mouse to a life-threatening extent.''

Skipper wrote a classic paper in 1964 detailing the inverse relationship between the amount of cancer in the body and its curability. If he gave small doses of drugs, fewer cancer cells were killed, but if he gave large doses, he could cure some of the animals with the drugs then available. Howard was disappointed at how hard it was to persuade many doctors that the dose-response relationship was critical. When Howard presented this clear-cut data, even many years later, some doctor would always stand up in the audience and say that he could do as well when treating patients with low doses of chemotherapy.

At the same time, as Howard would be the first to admit, the problem was more complex than the dose-response relationship would suggest. ''I will sadly admit that we tried half-blindly for fifteen years or so to cure this transplantable mouse leukemia with no success. True, we could treat the leukemic animals and increase their survival time, but during those fifteen lean years we buried an extraordinary number of mice that died of our experimental disease in spite of our efforts to save them.''

He found that cancerous cells fall into three growth states: those that are rapidly dividing, those that are temporarily nondividing but able to revert back, and those that are no longer capable of division. Drugs turned out to be most effective on the cells that are in rapid-division phase. The cells in the temporarily nondividing phase are partly or completely untouched by the drugs. (In the final phase, the cells die on their own without dividing and thus do not concern the cancer researcher.) The greater the fraction of cells that are dividing, the greater the chance of killing them. In mouse leukemia, and in childhood leukemia (and some fast-growing human tumors), the cancerous cells all divide rapidly and are very vulnerable to the drugs during division.

"But we knew from clinical studies going on in parallel that, with a single drug, you could get remissions in patients with acute lymphocytic leukemia, but then they would relapse. Patients weren't able to tolerate sufficient drug to kill all the cells in the first place, and the ones that grew back were resistant to chemotherapy, just as we were seeing in our mouse leukemia studies. All of us came to the conclusion that drug resistance was the step that was limiting our ability to make further progress in cancer chemotherapy." This realization propelled research on combinations of drugs both in Skipper's mouse labs and on Frei and Freireich's leukemia wards at the National Cancer Institute.

"This is kind of complex when you try to work it out in practice. When you alter the dose or frequency of administration of one drug within a combination of drugs, you may at the same time alter the effects of one or all the others. This all gets rather complicated and leads to the conclusion that, under certain circumstances, it may be better to use two drugs than four or five if the dose has to be reduced to below what's optimal for the most important drugs. Since it obviously isn't possible to do all the testing in humans, we must make very careful approximations based on animal experimentation. For example, we discovered that two drugs, cytosine arabinoside and 6-thioguanine, both antimetabolites, worked well in adults with acute myelogenous leukemia after we first modeled them in animals. I still feel that we don't know how best to use combinations of drugs in clinical situations, how best to use the mustard types of agents versus the antimetabolites, and how to select the best dose intensities to get the maximum effect in resistant cancers."

Although Howard recognizes how much remains to be learned, he still gets impatient with the physicians and scientists who cast doubt on the whole endeavor. "I remember the perennial pessimists who would sleep through or fail to understand reports of stepwise progress and then tell us:

- You will never discover drugs that will be useful in treating cancers.
- Yes, chemotherapy may cause temporary remissions in childhood leukemias and some other lymphomas, but it will never achieve cures.
- Maybe chemotherapy will cure some leukemias and lymphomas but it will never cure 'solid tumors'; choriocarcinoma in women and Wilms' tumor are different from all others. [The patients outlived these critics.]
- Maybe drugs when used with surgery will increase the remission duration and possibly the cure rate of disseminated breast cancer (in premenopausal women), but that is different. Surgery does most of the job. This approach will never be useful against most disseminated cancers. [This comment is still heard today, but not from those who have thought seriously about the mistakes unwittingly made in the past, the reasons why chemotherapy fails when it fails, and the approaches that will be required to reduce chemotherapeutic failures.]

"Pity the poor chemists, biologists, experimental pharmacologists, and mouse doctors. We heard all the dismal, dogmatic predictions and then got berated further by the clinicians. Gentle remarks like these (not necessarily verbatim) still ring in my ears:

- The drugs you dummies come up with are no darn good. They are too toxic. Why don't you discover a penicillin for cancer? (That is a good idea.)
- When I make my rounds and find my beds filled with mice, then, and only then, will I pay any attention to what those experimentalists think. (I never have been able to think of a proper reply to this one except, 'Good day.')
- A dose-response relationship may be seen in treating animal cancers, but I can do just as well with low-dose chemotherapy as with aggressive chemotherapy.
- Fancy scheduling isn't important in treating human cancers with drugs. I can do just as well with a daily dose schedule as with any other.
- Combination chemotherapy? The available drugs are too toxic even when given singly.
- An inverse relationship between amount of cancer and curability with drugs? Balderdash!"

Over time, these kinds of barbs at animal research were largely disproven by Howard Skipper, Frank Schabel, Abe Goldin, Lloyd Law, and other "mouse doctors."

For Howard Skipper, the "future of cancer research does not look bleak at all, if the younger generation of scientists and physicians can avoid some of the pitfalls that many of us have fallen in over the past thirty years or so. There's no better way to avoid those pitfalls than to look at all the available data, clinical and basic alike. Both have much to tell us if only we ask the right questions."

As for his own life in cancer research, Howard "would like to think that some of the things that our group has done may have helped shed light on why cancer treatment sometimes succeeds and sometimes fails and how the success rate might significantly increase." He looks back with pleasure on his personal life, his forty-five-year marriage to Margaret T. Edwards, and their two children. "I could not imagine a happier life together." He gave up playing golf to avoid the frustration of no longer being able to break eighty, but continues to cut gems as a hobby. "I suppose my real hobby is coming into the office and looking for some insights in our old data. There are so many wonderful experiments that are still trying to tell us something. I don't have any regrets. If I had to do it all over again, there are very few things I'd want to do differently."

CHAPTER 11

James Holland, M.D.

The whole of science is nothing more than a refinement of everyday thinking.
—Albert Einstein

If you found Frei and Freireich an interesting coincidence of names at NCI, think of Doctors Jim and Jimmie Holland. Jim, who is a key player in the leukemia story, is director of the Cancer Center at Mount Sinai Hospital in New York; Jimmie is chief of psychiatry at Memorial Sloan-Kettering Cancer Center. Jim is a world expert on the chemotherapy of cancer, Jimmie on the role of the mind in patients with cancer. The two members of this unique husband-wife team complement each other in professional interests as much as they contrast in style and demeanor; theirs is a highly successful model for marriage. Jim's story is essential not only for understanding progress in leukemia research but for documenting the little steps along the way in changing the public health consequences of acute leukemia.

Behind Dr. James Holland's desk stands a sculpture of great beauty that depicts the biblical story of Abraham and his son Isaac. The boy has just been mercifully retrieved from the altar of sacrifice, and the father holds his child urgently close in a gesture that is a perfect expression of love. The sculpture is the work of an American artist who lost his child to leukemia. He gave the casting of the two poignant figures to the Leukemia Society of America. The society adopted it as the symbol for its "Return of the Child" award and made its first presentation to Dr. Holland. It is an honor of which he is extremely proud, for it represents recognition of his many years heading the most successful long-term cooperative group studies of leukemia chemotherapy.

210

Jim grew up in Morristown, New Jersey. His father was a county judge. His mother, an exceptionally intelligent woman, had to drop out of school after the eighth grade because her mother had died and she had to raise the rest of the family.

Jim's parents decided they wanted a large family after they suffered the death of their second child, a toddler who was accidentally poisoned by his grandmother's pills. After the tragedy they had three more sons (Jim was the third of the four surviving brothers) and adopted a daughter.

Jim's father, an intellectual in the traditional sense of the word, would give his children rewards for learning poems. In elementary school, in turn, Jim consistently won prizes for earning the highest grades and loved the books of poetry that were frequently his reward. Jim's father had a wonderful command of language and harbored the hope that Jim would become a lawyer. Although Jim followed a different path, his stentorian voice and ready speech on any subject may well find their origins in his father's example. Jim and two of his brothers became doctors; the fourth became an engineer.

Jim went to Morristown High School, as his father had. Thanks to his high grades, he skipped his freshman year. Despite being the youngest student in his class, he did very well, met girls, and generally had a good time. At his father's request, he went off to military school for his junior year of high school, attracted by the thought of having a horse to ride every day and the fact that his oldest brother had gone to the same institution and had been captain of the troop. Once there, however, Jim disliked it intensely. He missed his freedom and resented the hypocrisy of the headmaster.

Jim told his father that the military academy was a "rich man's reform school" and refused to go back. He returned to Morristown High School, where he was much happier, and became salutatorian of his senior class.

Jim enrolled at Princeton University in 1941. With no idea of what he would eventually do, he took courses in biology, chemistry, politics, English, French, and mathematics.

"I took a freshman course in biology from a wonderful teacher. In high school biology we had done frog dissections and learned about plant biology, but to see living one-celled animals, to see them ingesting their food, and to see their amoeboid movement was extremely interesting. The mitotic apparatus at the tip of an onion root was fascinating to me."

On December 7, 1941, Jim hitchhiked from a weekend at home back to campus, turned on the radio, and heard the unbelievable news of the bombing of Pearl Harbor. The next day, December 8, Princeton began mobilizing its people. The university president, Harold Dodds, assembled the entire student body in the largest auditorium on the campus and pleaded with them not to resign and enlist, pointing out that the army and navy had already told the school that what they needed were leaders and officers. Dodds said that Princeton would immediately expand its training of officers. The college went into continuous session, and Jim spent all of the next two years in Princeton. He was inducted into the navy and assigned to Princeton as a V-12 student.

Jim backed into the decision to go to medical school. Judge Holland would have preferred law school, but he had already approved of medical school for Jim's older brother. A career in pure science seemed ruled out by Jim's problems with calculus and a highly mathematical physical chemistry course, yet he had enjoyed his biology and biological chemistry classes and had the prerequisites for medical school. Even though he felt no passionate calling to medicine at the time, he nonetheless sent in his applications.

Inevitably, the first question in interviews was: "Do you feel you're too young to go to medical school?" In January 1944 Jim was only eighteen years old, yet fully prepared academically for medical school. Because the medical school course was also accelerated in wartime, it was possible that Jim could graduate still too young to obtain a license and practice.

Jim always studied hard in college. The strenuous accelerated program suited him. "I've never met anybody who in working to his full capacity doesn't have to work hard: if someone is to accomplish all that his natural endowment allows, then he has to work. No one is so brilliant that he or she can do their best without working to the limit of his/her own competence. I've always been capable of studying for hours at a time without complaint. I just enjoy learning and working at things that are intellectually stimulating."

Jim accepted the first offer he got, from Columbia's College of Physicians and Surgeons. Despite his original lack of conviction, medical school turned out to be a fabulous success. His first year, he had the good luck to have as his physiology instructor Dr. Alfred Gellhorn, a remarkable man. Then at the peak of his career, Gellhorn aroused Jim's interest in endocrinology and cancer. Jim selected for his class research project the subject of the prostate gland. Dr. Charles Huggins, later to win a Nobel Prize for his work, had just reported on the effect of castration on the prostate gland in dogs, and workers at Columbia were examining the importance of enzymes made by prostate cells as markers of prostate cancer. Jim Holland went far beyond the requirements and wrote a full-scale thesis on which Gellhorn wrote "An A+. Because I have no corrections to make." He went on to ask a series of scientific questions that treated Jim like a colleague, not a mere freshman medical student.

Jim's path crossed Gellhorn's again in the second-year pharmacology course and in the third-year internal medicine course. Several years later, when Jim came back to New York City after his residency and military service, he worked for two years as chief resident and NIH research fellow under Gellhorn, who was now director of the Delafield Hospital, Columbia's cancer hospital in New York.

After graduation from Columbia Physicians and Surgeons, Jim did his internship and assistant residency at Columbia-Presbyterian Hospital, where he had another outstanding role model, Dr. Robert F. Loeb, whom he describes as "a giant of a man, one of the two or three brightest men I've ever met.

"Robert F. Loeb was a magnificent teacher; he was Jehovah incarnate for me. Once he asked the students what the x-ray and the clinical findings were for patients who had abscesses around the kidney. I knew, and the others didn't. Another time he was making rounds and encountered a patient with Guillain-Barré syndrome. He asked how one could distinguish this neurological disease from poliomyelitis, and I answered the question correctly. He didn't say anything to me but turned to the ward attending doctors and asked, 'Who trained this man?' When my immediate superior spoke up, Loeb shook his hand. And that was the nicest compliment that I think I'd ever had."

The reputation of the Columbia-Presbyterian Medical Service rose to great heights under the leadership of Dr. Loeb. Loeb's prodigious memory and knowledge of the research literature impressed Jim, but so did Loeb's concern for the people he was treating. Loeb was often called upon to examine profoundly sick patients, not just in the course of his normal rounds, but because these cases seemed too complicated for others to figure out what to do. Jim particularly remembers one boy who had empyema— pus in his chest. They'd stuck a needle into him and gotten out some foul-smelling material. The boy wanted to be left alone. He was in pain, whining, wasted, chronically ill, and afraid. The doctors asked Dr. Loeb to come and decide what to do. It was about 6:00 in the evening. His decision was given with absolute assurance, "Let the boy have a night's sleep and tomorrow open his chest." Jim comments, "I think that even today, looking back on it, I, too, would have said, 'We have to open his chest.' But Dr. Loeb had the wisdom to give the boy a little surcease from what was clearly more than the kid could stand. That was a wonderful example for us."

Although Loeb had no special interest in cancer, it was his continuing interest in Jim Holland that was responsible for Jim's ending up in oncology. "While I was serving in the army, Loeb sent me a handwritten letter which I still have, describing himself as the bad penny turning up again, but really wanted to know if I was coming back. I wrote that I'd love to come back, but couldn't promise because there was a rumor at that time that army doctors would be transferred from Europe to Korea. He wrote back saying he'd arrange something. When I went back in September 1951 he said, 'Everything's filled at Presbyterian Hospital, but somebody will drop out with psychiatric problems or tuberculosis, they always do, and then I'll call you back. In the meantime, why don't you go down to Delafield Hospital, the new cancer hospital we opened.' I did, and there was Alfred Gellhorn in charge of the Medical Service. That was a wonderful synthesis and synergy. A good fit. So, when Dr. Loeb called me back to say that he had a position open, I said, 'Thank you, Dr. Loeb, but I think I'll stay here.'

"Although Delafield was a first-rate cancer hospital, by specializing in that disease it wasn't in the mainstream for Columbia-Presbyterian Medical Center. Dr. Gellhorn gave as many grand rounds as possible at Presbyterian to keep Dr. Loeb and the rest of the medical service aware of the cancer program at Delafield.

The first Delafield case that Jim Holland presented was that of a child who had been treated with the drug aminopterin, the first successful antileukemic drug. Josephine was all of four years old and due to make a personal appearance at medical grand rounds in the big auditorium at Presbyterian Hospital. The semicircular amphitheater with brass railings was an intimidating setting.

"Because this child was coming from home, I bought a couple of balloons and tied them to the brass rail so I could give her balloons and entice her into the 'pit.' I had come to love this child, and she loved me. She came in and made a big hit, and the balloon decoration went over very successfully. David Segal, a senior professor of medicine and one of my teachers, paid me a wonderful compliment in the elevator going down when he said, 'Jim, you've mesmerized me.'

"Her remission was extremely meaningful to me, but by the same token, it was tragic when she relapsed and died. Her father was horribly grieved, because she was his only child. There was just unbelievable trauma for everybody concerned. I was only a resident at that time, and this was my first case of leukemia after I had come back from the army, and the first cancer patient that I put into remission.

"I've thought a lot about Josephine—and so many other patients as well. I recall the care that we took to manage her blood counts. We measured them frequently. This of course was before the days of platelet transfusion. We had the anguish of dealing with nosebleeds, gum bleeding, and bruises in the skin; and primitive antibiotics were all we had available then to treat infections. And she was only a child, a crying child."

Jim's failure to show similar sensitivity to his patient's feelings on another occasion brought down Dr. Loeb's wrath on him. The fact that Loeb by now regarded Jim as one of his "intellectual sons" probably gave extra strength to his rebuke. At morning rounds, Jim had given the history of a seventy-year-old black man, a small man with prostate cancer.

"When I presented his story, I referred to him as a 'case' and then referred to him as this 'seventy-year-old gent.' I didn't realize it at the time, but my language became the topic of Dr. Loeb's morning meeting with the residents the following day on the kind of disaffection a good man can get into—how outrageous it was to denigrate somebody by calling him a 'gent.' I got the word back from Dr. Gellhorn that Dr. Loeb had really laced into him about my unfeeling behavior for this black man in referring to him in what must have seemed like a supercilious and less than respectful way, as a 'gent.' Later on he laid it on me directly.

"I was absolutely devastated, because I didn't mean it in those terms. I don't see myself as being superior or thinking at the level of racial or class disparagement. But apparently it sounded like that. It took me a long while to get over that mistake. The point is that Dr. Loeb's motivation was correct. His feeling was that you treat patients with respect—all patients, no matter what.

"In many ways Loeb fulfilled the role of medical father to me, with a kind of detached, cool but involved paternal love. My own father was warm and involved. But then, Loeb had a hundred intellectual sons. I don't know where I ranked, and it doesn't matter. I ranked, and that's what counts. He took me on the path, and he approved."

At Delafield, Gellhorn immediately set Jim on the road to becoming a clinical researcher. Jim was given an independent research project on a new drug, EDTA (ethylene-diaminetetraacetic acid). Its ability to remove excessive calcium is sometimes a problem for patients with cancer. As Jim mastered the techniques of measuring calcium levels, catheterizing dogs to infuse the drug experimentally, and observing the drug's effects on cancer patients with excessive levels of calcium in their blood, he gained respect for the difficulties of doing basic biomedical research. He appreciated the generosity of senior researchers at other New York hospitals who shared with him their hard-won technical skills: "Your father, Dr. Daniel Laszlo, and his wife, Dr. Herta Spencer, at Montefiore were the only people in the country studying EDTA in patients with high serum calcium. Your father couldn't have been nicer to me. He taught me a great deal about various methods of measuring calcium. Everything about the project was open, and he continued to advise me. It was really a very warm and important experience in science for me." He was equally grateful to the great pharmacologist Alfred Gilman, who taught him how to infuse dogs with EDTA for a complex experiment on the interplay between parathyroid hormone secretion and blood calcium levels.

Jim also learned the hard but salutary lesson that one can do good experiments, yet still get inconclusive results. He had wanted to find out whether a sudden precipitous drop in blood calcium levels triggered by a dose of EDTA would stimulate parathyroid hormone secretion and in turn stimulate a rise in serum calcium to protect the body from dangerously low levels of calcium. In exactly half of his twenty experimental dogs, the drug-induced drop in calcium did indeed trigger the hormone. But in the other half, it did not. Jim got conflicting advice about how to handle this ambivalent result of a year's hard work. Gellhorn told him, "You shouldn't publish that because it doesn't prove anything." Gilman, however, said, "You should publish that because it will keep someone else from doing it." Jim's paper was rejected by the *Journal of General Physiology*, and, disappointed, he never sent it out again.

Another research project instigated by Gellhorn had equally inconclusive results, but its very inconclusiveness was revealing. "Dr. Gellhorn had never believed (nor has anybody else as far as I can tell) Dr. Sidney Farber's assertion that the reason he came to use aminopterin, an antifolate, was that, in giving folate products, the course of leukemia was accelerated. Gellhorn said, 'If that's so, boy, here's a new folate drug, citrovorum factor, that's even farther along in the metabolic scheme. Let's treat patients with it. We'll see what happens.' I must have treated twenty patients at Delafield with it: in ten of them, white blood cell counts rose, and in ten, the counts fell. We finally concluded that we hadn't really seen anything to confirm that giving folates exacerbated leukemia."

Despite the lack of publishable results, Jim had relished his taste of research and eagerly acted on Gellhorn's advice that he apply for a job at the National Cancer Institute's Clinical Center, which was due to open in 1953. Jim's personal circumstances also made a move to a better-paying job desirable. During his senior year of medical school he had married a young woman whose interests turned out to have little in common with his. Now after seven years of marriage and one child, Jim and his wife had gotten a divorce. The $4,000 a year NIH fellowship he had at Delafield would not be enough to support his ex-wife and daughter.

Gellhorn put in a good word with G. Burroughs Mider, a protein chemist and tumor physiologist who was clinical director of NCI. Mider, in turn, arranged for Jim to have an interview at Bethesda with Murray Shear, the father of tumor pharmacology.

"I went to the old National Cancer Institute research building in Bethesda, and there was Murray Shear with his Puck-like manner, a wise fellow, working on mice with cancer. He was studying the effects of a lipopolysaccharide called Shear's polysaccharide, a chemical that was extracted from the cell wall of the bacteria Serratia. He had found it to have anticancer properties in animals. In the particular experiment prior to my arrival he had given a lethal injection of the chemical, because he had a dead mouse on his hands. And he said to me, 'Autopsy that mouse. Find out why it died.' I was there for a job interview and he asked me to autopsy a mouse! I said, 'I've never autopsied a mouse before. I've never worked with mice.' He said, 'Good, fine. That'll be even better.'"

Jim was hired and, thanks to his interest and little bit of experience, became chief of chemotherapy under the chief of medicine, Dr. Leonard Fenninger, and hence NCI's senior chemotherapist. Jim was at NCI for only seventeen months, from July 1953 through November 1954, but his tenure there had long-lasting consequences for him, for NCI's leukemia program, and for leukemia research internationally.

Of all the people Jim met at NCI, the two that impressed him the most were Dr. Roy Hertz, a very experienced senior scientist who headed the endocrinology program, and Dr. Lloyd Law, an outstanding animal experimentalist. Jim's previous work on hormones made him interested in Hertz's experiments with aminopterin, because Hertz had shown that the antifolate drug interfered with the development of oviducts in chicks. That suggested that the drug might work on two fronts: interrupting the cooperation between enzymes and vitamins that speed metabolic reactions *and* affecting the hormonal regulation of tissue development. Hertz's work alerted Jim to the importance of considering all the modes of action that an anticancer drug might evince.

Jim met Lloyd Law soon after coming to NCI. Law had been preparing a presentation about his work for NIH's board of directors. Since he was not a physician, he appreciated Jim's offer to help with the interpretation of the clinical aspects of the research. As they met several times a week for a month, Jim got a close look at some of the best recent experimental chemotherapy on animals and made a lasting friend. Law had used a purine analog (8-azaguanine) with aminopterin in combination to treat animal leukemia—perhaps the first time anyone had tried the experiment of combining anticancer drugs.

By mid-1953 two other drugs had shown promise and were available for study: the purine analog, 6-MP, and the improved derivative of aminopterin, methotrexate. With Law's help and advice, Jim started testing a combination of 6-MP and methotrexate. He began with the proposition that if you can put a third of your patients into remission with methotrexate, and if you can put a third of your patients into remission with 6-MP, then one-ninth of the patients ought to respond especially well to both drugs. And among that ninth, some might be cured. Expressing this another way, suppose that thirty-three out of a hundred leukemic children would go into remission with either methotrexate or 6-MP. Achieving such a remission with one drug means that although the vast majority of leukemic cells have been killed, there will be a residual minority of cells that ultimately will multiply and cause a relapse. But if a third of these thirty-three patients were also sensitive to the second drug, the leukemic cells in these eleven patients would be so few in number and so inhibited that cures might even be possible. Jim's protocols for leukemia therapy at the National Cancer Institute treated all comers, children and adults alike, with a combination of 6-MP and methotrexate, the dosage calculated on the basis of weight.

In those early days at NCI, there were no rules or even established practice regarding how much evidence you needed from animal studies before trying out a new therapy on patients. They were making it up as they went along, those pioneers in clinical research. To Jim, Law's theoretical arguments for combining drugs and Law's results with mice using, so to speak, chemical rough drafts of 6-MP and methotrexate were ample justification for making that combination his standard treatment for NCI's leukemia patients. NCI's first clinical director, Dr. Mider, was mildly distressed that the 6-MP/methotrexate combination had not been tested in animals first, so he enlisted a pharmacologist, Dr. Abraham Goldin, to do a series of experiments with various doses and schedules of the combination on leukemic mice. From then on the interplay of animal studies and clinical studies became much tighter in leukemia research, and the amount of testing required in animals before taking a drug to patients became much more extensive.

In the fall of 1954, the newly expanded Roswell Park Memorial Cancer Institute in Buffalo offered Jim the post of Chief of Medicine. The job of running the inpatient service was a plum for so young a physician: Jim was only twenty-eight. It meant the chance to build a clinical research program from the ground up. And the pay was good—$11,300 a year compared with NCI's $7600. The pay raise enabled him to marry Dr. Jimmie Holland, whose expertise in the psychosocial side of cancer treatment complemented his own. Together they had five children over the next eight years.

Another attraction of Roswell Park was the strong commitment on the part of its director, Dr. George Moore, to cancer research. Moore, who had been appointed two years before (at the age of thirty-two) to make the institute a strong research facility, was a remarkable scientist and physician in his own right: he was the first person to grow human leukemia cells in tissue culture and made important advances in growing many types of cancer cells in the test tube. As an administrator, he had a talent for recruiting first-rate clinicians and researchers to Roswell Park: Jim Holland,

Donald Pinkel to head pediatrics (where he began his work on radiation therapy for leukemia patients), and other notable experts such as Joseph Sokal, David Pressman, and Chuck Nichol. As two strong personalities, Moore and Holland frequently came into conflict, but their mutual respect for each other's abilities carried the day: "There was no question about it, Moore was bright, very self-assured, arrogant, and authoritarian in many ways. Because I have never liked arbitrary authority exercised over me (once a Princeton professor said to me, 'Well, Holland, everybody knows you are an anarchist anyhow!'), he and I were cool and distant on many things. But we were also able to work together when it had to do with pure brain power, because he appreciated my intellect, and I had considerable appreciation for his ability to get things done."

It often takes a "critical mass" of talented people to move an institution and a field. Roswell Park now had this in leukemia—especially with two dynamic people like Jim Holland and Don Pinkel. Jim points to Don as having made a major contribution on how to better calculate drug dosages for children, a perennial problem in making the conversion from information gained with adults. As we have seen, while Don was convalescing from polio he worked out the concept that dosage shouldn't be calculated on the basis of body weight—critical functions like bone marrow toxicity related better to dosage calculated on the basis of body surface area. Jim also notes Don's contributions to the use of chemotherapy prior to the use of surgery for sarcomas in children and to his early studies with Walter Murphy at Roswell on treating leukemia with radiation therapy to the brain. The latter took hold later, when Don headed up the program at St. Jude and changed the course of the disease when he increased the dosage.

Jim's move to Buffalo coincided with a change higher up at NCI. G. Burroughs Mider moved to the position of scientific director at the Clinical Center. His replacement as clinical director was a newcomer, Gordon Zubrod. During Zubrod's tour of NCI, Mider introduced him to Jim, who had only a month left in Bethesda.

"Zubrod couldn't have been nicer. He said to me, 'I don't have a program in leukemia. Would you mind if we continued your program after you leave?' And I said, 'I would be delighted. If you continue to do that, then I'll continue to do it in Buffalo.' " That brief meeting was the unofficial start of collaborative leukemia studies involving NCI, Roswell Park, and the Buffalo General Hospital.

In Buffalo, Jim continued treating leukemia patients with 6-MP and methotrexate. By telephone, he and Gordon Zubrod kept on discussing their work and the news from other researchers around the country. After Tom Frei was recruited, Jim paid a visit to Bethesda, probably early in 1955, and sat down with Tom and Gordon to discuss future research. Zubrod thought it was time to conduct a comparative trial, perhaps comparing the combination of two drugs against a single drug.

Jim argued that such an experiment would be unethical, because they already knew that the combination had the potential for cure while everyone treated with single drugs had died. Gordon agreed that no one should do anything he believed to be unethical and said that, because it was Jim's program in the first place, they ought to accept Jim's view. Instead, they should design the study in such a way that it was ethically acceptable to all. Abe Goldin's work with mouse leukemia suggested that intermittent higher doses of methotrexate were more effective in inducing and extending remissions than lower doses daily. So Zubrod, Frei, and Holland came to a compromise: all the patients in this first comparative study would stay on a daily dose of 6-MP, but half would get the regular daily dose of methotrexate that Jim had been prescribing all along while the other half got tripled doses of methotrexate every third day.

"It is of interest that we didn't then have any real understanding that maybe what we should have done was to see if patients could take even more methotrexate when they took it every third day. We didn't do a feasibility or pilot study (as would be needed today) to see if that was possible. The study might have been a great success if we'd used ten times the dose, but we used only three times the dose. By the time that first study was published in 1956, we had become more formally organized, and a biostatistician, Marvin Schneiderman, worked with us on the design of comparative studies. Tom Frei had much more time and resources at the National Cancer Institute than I had at Roswell Park, so he took on the administrative chores and consulting with the statistician." Thanks to Gordon Zubrod at NCI, this was the first cooperative program involving Roswell Park, the National Cancer Institute, and the Buffalo General Hospital.

"Tom Frei recruited a number of other prominent hematologists from various hospitals to participate in the cooperative study. Together we showed there was no significant difference between the two programs of administering methotrexate in combination with daily 6-MP. The second study was then designed to compare the combination against a sequential plan in which one drug was given first, and then the other."

Over the next half-dozen years, the Acute Leukemia Group B expanded to bring in hematologists and patients from other institutions around the country. It concentrated first on comparing the combination of methotrexate and 6-MP given daily versus three times the dose but given every third day. (In retrospect, Jim knows that much larger doses could have been tolerated when the combination was given every third day.)

"In 1963, Tom Frei was gaining more duties at the Cancer Institute and I was now comfortably ensconced at Roswell. Tom wanted out of his administrative role as chairman of the cooperative group Acute Leukemia Group B, so an election was held. The two candidates were J Freireich and me, and I must say there was some apprehension on the part of a few that J, who is even less conventional than I am, might win; but indeed in an election (which wasn't rigged), I did win. So I moved the headquarters from Washington to Buffalo, which amounted to moving a couple of paper cartons."

Although the point of the cooperative group was to assemble enough patients to give statistical validity to therapeutic claims, Jim found—as Frei had before him—that getting creative physician-scientists to cooperate was not so easy. Just before the end of Tom's tenure, J Freireich had pulled out of the group in order to create the VAMP program where the new compound vincristine was used in conjunction with three older drugs at once. The cooperative group under Holland's lead opted for more deliberate studies of vincristine's effectiveness, with one or two drugs at a time.

While granting that Freireich got "enormous mileage" out of the VAMP program, Jim Holland believes that the cooperative group's Protocol 6307 (that is, the seventh study in 1963) also obtained valuable results. "The protocol's spaced dosing—vincristine and prednisone given to induce remission followed by daily or twice-weekly methotrexate—yielded a four-fold increase in the duration of the remissions, because we could increase the methotrexate dose eightfold. At the time, the beneficial effect was ascribed more to the schedule of drug administration than to the dose, but in retrospect, and judging from some others' studies, dose intensity may have been the critical factor; the way we gave the drug was just a convenient way to get the dose in. There was a very impressive difference in the remission durations. That study was the first real change in the effectiveness of folic antagonists on childhood leukemia since the discovery of the drugs in Farber's original report and Burchenal's confirmation of their activity."

Jim's position as chair of the cooperative group gave him no immunity from criticism from its other members. For example, he was bitterly disappointed when a sequential program he proposed in 1963 was turned down by the group, primarily because Tom Frei spoke against it.

"The study that we did was excellent, but it would have been better had it been done my way, I think." To Jim, the problem with combination chemotherapy was that each drug got used in less than its regular full dose. His solution was to give each drug in full dose, but in a sequential fashion: first use drug A in full dose, then B, C, and D to kill off the remaining cells sequentially. In particular, the design that he wanted to try in study 6313 was vincristine and prednisone administration to achieve a quick remission followed sequentially by courses of cyclophosphamide, 6-MP, methotrexate, and a new drug, BCNU. (BCNU, bis-chloronitrosourea, was another experimental drug being tested at the time. Its principal attributes were that it crossed the blood vessel/membrane barrier into the brain and had a very different chemical structure.) After each step, the drugs would be stopped for a random sample of patients to measure how long the unmaintained remission would last; then the scientists could calculate how much leukemic cell killing had occurred.

"Tom argued, even though he wasn't participating, that such a design would be too complex for the group to follow. It taught me a lesson. You really shouldn't have a voice at the table unless you're a participant." The actual study was still quite complicated: after vincristine and prednisone induced remission, the patient got three courses of methotrexate, or three courses of 6-MP, or three doses of cyclophosphamide, or the sequence of cyclophosphamide, 6-MP, and methotrexate. Half of the people who received the cyclophosphamide/6-MP/methotrexate sequence were also given BCNU as a way to test its efficacy.

"The outcome was that the sequence of vincristine, prednisone, cyclophosphamide, 6-MP, methotrexate, and BCNU gave a longer unmaintained remission than did the NCI VAMP program, and that's published. But we didn't have the strong press reaction that characterized announcement of the VAMP data, and it never had the same impact on the field. Over the subsequent twenty-five years we continued to work on the general concept of sequential drug administration.

"The arguments among members of the cooperative groups occasionally had unexpected payoffs. A brash young NCI investigator named Ed Henderson came to a group meeting once (he had never previously been to a meeting as far as I can remember), saw this program of 6-MP and methotrexate and cyclophosphamide, and said, 'My God, those doses are dangerous, you're going to kill children with those doses of methotrexate and you're going to kill patients with those doses of cyclophosphamide.' So, deferentially, because groups always go to the least common denominator, we cut the doses of methotrexate from 15 milligrams per square meter of body surface area to 12 per square meter and cut the dose of cyclophosphamide from 1,000 to 600. And we treated another six to ten patients on each of these new lower doses without changing the patients who were already started on 15 or 1,000. But nobody died with the original methotrexate dose, and nobody died on the cyclophosphamide; Henderson's Cassandra pronouncements fizzled. We went back to the original doses.

"When we made the final analyses on these cases, the results in the group treated with 12 milligrams per square meter of methotrexate, as Henderson had advocated, were significantly inferior to the group treated with 15 milligrams per square meter. It was a small number of cases, but it was inferior enough to set us on the road to our next study, looking at responses to different methotrexate doses, using courses of 12, 15, or 18 per square meter. But, remarkably, the group treated with 1,000 milligrams per square meter of cyclophosphamide was inferior to the 600: the *lower* dose of cyclophosphamide was superior to the higher dose. This suggested that the high dose of cyclophosphamide was probably suppressing the immune response of the children. We properly interpreted these disparate results, so that ultimately we got more information out of the study by these circuitous serendipitous excursions than we would have by using our original plan." Curiously, Dr. Henderson later succeeded Dr. Holland at Roswell Park when Jim moved to Mount Sinai in 1973.

"The next serious effort to study methotrexate started in 1966 and may have been the finest study done by our group. Study 6601 again induced remissions with vincristine and prednisone and then randomly assigned patients to receive methotrexate at 12, 15, or 18 milligrams per square meter daily in five-day courses. One set of patients was treated with just three courses of methotrexate, as in the original study, and one set got eight months of five-day courses. The rationale for the eight months of treatment was important. This was based on estimates by us and others of the body burden of leukemic cells in a child—the total amount of leukemic cells contained in the bone marrow, blood, lymph nodes, spleen, and elsewhere: about one kilogram (2.2 lbs.) of leukemic tissue in a child with florid leukemia."

Jim had calculated that had they kept on with the methotrexate killing for 120 days, instead of for only three courses (fifteen days), they would have eradicated the whole population of leukemic cells. To stay on the safe side, they allowed for an error of a factor of two in their calculations, and designed the next program to include 240 days (8 months) of intensive methotrexate courses at doses of 12, 15, or 18 milligrams per square meter. Thus the study compared three treatment programs: (1) three courses after the vincristine, prednisone induction; (2) eight months of courses, with vincristine and prednisone reinforcement interspersed every third course; (3) the twice-weekly methotrexate maintenance regimen, which they had proved in 1963 to be a good program. With the three courses, just one child was cured; but 18 percent were cured with eight months of courses, and 30 percent were cured with the eight months of courses plus vincristine and prednisone reinforcement. It took this kind of meticulous clinical research on the effectiveness of different dosage schedules to begin the quantum leap in curing the disease.

Jim continued to chair the cooperative group for eighteen years altogether, despite the strains caused by strong personalities among its members and despite incidents in his own life that might well have persuaded another person to step down from the demanding task. In 1966 he endured a terrible accident when a horse he was riding with his four-year-old daughter reared, fell back, and crushed him underneath. "I can still see myself consciously realizing what was happening and throwing my daughter out of the way (she was unharmed) and then hearing my pelvis crunch as the horse fell down on me." Fortunately he made a full recovery. Ten years later, four years after he had moved from Roswell Park to head the new Department of Neoplastic Diseases at New York's Mount Sinai School of Medicine, Jim had a heart attack on a commuter train and ended up in Mount Sinai's emergency room. He had bypass surgery several years after that. Yet, all the while, the cooperative group kept working—ultimately growing to include more than two hundred researchers from about thirty institutions in Denmark, France, Switzerland, South Africa, Canada, and across the United States. The stability of Jim's leadership, his ability to make all the members of the group feel that they were contributing something valuable, the deep bonds of personal friendship and mutual trust that linked many of the researchers, and the signs of steady progress held the group together longer than any other cooperative group in cancer.

The cooperative group's emphasis was always on continuing studies of acute lymphocytic leukemia, but it expanded its scope to work on other forms of cancer whenever animal models or the leukemia results seemed to provide a lead. Similarly, group members exploited ideas from research on other cancers whenever they could. The decision to use methotrexate in five-day courses in the 6601 protocol, for example, was based on NCI research on choriocarcinoma.

Jim Holland had paid attention to choriocarcinoma ever since 1956, when he had heard from a friend that someone in Dr. Roy Hertz's group at NCI had used methotrexate to treat a woman with the disease and had seen a good response. When a woman with metastatic choriocarcinoma came to Roswell Park soon afterwards, Jim decided to try methotrexate with her. She responded so dramatically that Jim hastened to report her case in print—even before M. C. Li, Roy Hertz, and D. B. Spencer published their first paper on the subject in 1956. Jim's patient became the second-longest-surviving cancer patient to be cured by chemotherapy—alive and still well after more than thirty-seven years.

Given this experience, Jim naturally took a deep interest in the story of choriocarcinoma research and treatment, the first clear-cut success story in cancer therapy. Unlike J Freireich, who gives all the credit to M. C. Li, Jim Holland thinks more recognition ought to go to Dr. Paul Condit, the chemotherapist-pharmacologist who actually first gave extremely high single doses of methotrexate to choriocarcinoma patients. As Jim Holland tells the story, Condit, working with Abe Goldin on leukemic mice, needed to follow up with studies on humans. He asked Dr. Li if he could treat patients who were not being actively treated on Dr. Hertz's service, and Li allowed him to try methotrexate on some patients with choriocarcinoma.

Li had been measuring the levels of human choriogonadotrophic hormone (HCG) in these patients (with an eye to eventually removing the pituitary gland, a source of the hormone, to see if that affected the growth of the cancer).

When Condit gave the patients methotrexate, Li saw their HCG hormone levels drop. Sensing that the patients were improving, Li then refused to let Condit continue with his experiments and instead gave patients the extremely high doses of 25 milligrams a day (for five consecutive days) himself. Li's paper on his results thanked Condit in a footnote for his contributions to the research. Jim comments: "It's true that Li recognized the fall in HCG, which was the critical observation. However, the actual giving of methotrexate to the patient was not related to the mouse experiments by Goldin on the best way to shrink tumors with methotrexate. It was serendipity. Condit should have gotten a larger share of the credit and didn't. After Li left NCI, Hertz pursued the refinement of the therapy and ran with the ball, establishing the curative regime."

Still a third version of the story, and the most common one, credits Dr. Hertz himself with the cure of choriocarcinoma. According to this interpretation, Hertz had seen how folic acid antagonists prevented the development of the chick oviduct; it was therefore clear to him that such drugs would also act on the placenta's growth and placenta-derived cancer (that is, choriocarcinoma). In any case, as director of NCI's Endocrinology Division and the person in charge of the choriocarcinoma patients and the research on them, Hertz's name went first on most of the papers published about the research, and he got the recognition.

Today there is no way of sorting out these stories—and who knows if there are not other versions as well. Two key figures, Hertz and Li, are no longer alive. Even though I myself was on the spot at the time—working briefly on the Endocrine Service as an NCI fellow and treating some of those patients—I cannot guess how the proper credit ought to be allocated. After all, no one there at the time was aware that these patients were being cured.

Indeed, no one would be sure for years whether choriocarcinoma had been cured. The comparable question was even harder to settle for leukemia. For Jim, as an individual researcher and as head of a cooperative group in the early days of leukemia treatment, the dilemma that accompanied every promising protocol, every remission was: how could you know whether the chemotherapy had really done the trick? Leukemia had no measuring stick to mark the total destruction of cancerous cells, unlike choriocarcinoma, where the level of HCG hormone told you roughly how many cancer cells were left. Bone marrow tests and blood cells could only tell you so much. Like Freireich and Frei, Jim Holland came to the difficult conclusion that the only way to be sure was to stop treatment.

CANCER AND LEUKEMIA GROUP B
Acute lymphocytic leukemia survival in children under 20
1956-1980

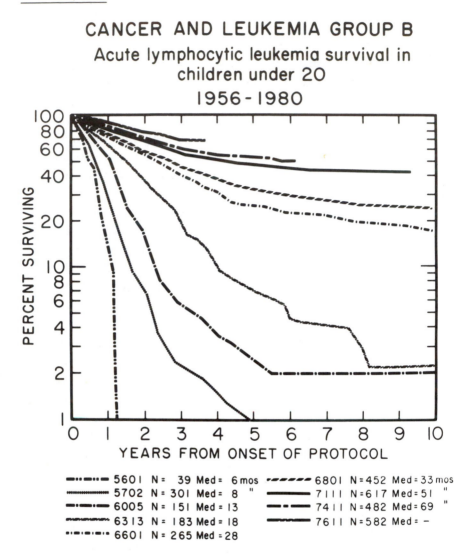

4. Incremental improvement in survival of children treated according to protocols conducted by the Acute Leukemia Group B, also called Cancer and Leukemia Group B. The first protocol of 1956 (5601) included thirty-nine patients (N = 39); the final one depicted here started in 1976 (7611) and included 582 patients. The median survival of each study is indicated on the right of each legend—it was six months for the first protocol and the median had not been reached for the last protocol by the time of analysis in 1980. *(Kindly furnished by Dr. James Holland for the ALGB.)*

"I must say that the decision to end treatment for children in remission, whether it was after three courses or eight months of maintenance chemotherapy, got venomous criticism from Sidney Farber, who thought that to deliberately allow children to relapse was unethical. Farber was a titan, and his rebuke did concern us. But there is absolutely no way to discover the effectiveness of experimental treatment except by stopping treatment."

The data on how many patients survived for how long before relapsing were critical. After the first couple of protocols, Jim prepared charts of survival curves; and again after the first half-dozen protocols; and kept on doing so all the time he was in charge of the cooperative group. Each year, the charts told the story: more and more leukemia patients were living long after their treatments were stopped. It was fair to say that chemotherapy had cured them.

"The reward of creativity is the satisfaction of seeing one's creation work, but seeing it oneself isn't the only thing one savors, it's appreciation by others. If you don't get appreciated, you may indeed be equally proud; but there are very few people who aren't influenced by society, as such. Society ultimately donates rewards and other satisfactions by their reception of somebody's work or status. Is it important to have things like the Nobel Prize? Sure. And it's a great satisfaction to have that prize, the first Return of the Child Award ever given. But even without the prizes and the statues, the concept of being first and demonstrating it to one's peers and competitors is very rewarding in its own right."

For Jim, that reward came in the words of one of his former students, Dr. Bill Peters, at a conference at Duke around 1985: "He pointed out that the real achievement is not to have drawn the chart, but to have conceived the program and to have taken the steps *before* it was known that the line was going to represent improved survival. We were mighty pleased at that!"

CHAPTER 12

Donald Pinkel, M.D.: Culmination

There is not enough darkness in all the world to put out the light of even one small candle.
—*Robert Alden*

"From its start, St. Jude Children's Research Hospital in Memphis, Tennessee, took childhood leukemia research and treatment as its special mission. You might wonder why Memphis—hardly a mecca of medical research. It began with Danny Thomas. He got his professional start in Chicago, but it was slow going at first. He vowed that, if he succeeded, he would build a shrine to St. Jude. By the mid-1950s he was doing well and he consulted Cardinal Stritch, who had been very interested in medicine. As a young priest in Memphis, Stritch had seen children suffering, and he advised Danny to build a children's hospital there instead: 'There are plenty of shrines.' The local medical groups resisted, however, and the project was on the rocks. Danny arranged for an all-star benefit, the likes of which Memphis had never seen. At the end, in an emotional appeal, he asked doctors to come forward to aid him." Two distinguished physicians, Gilbert Levy and Lemuel Diggs, came forward. They subsequently advised that the focus be a research center for children with catastrophic illnesses like leukemia. In Dr. Donald Pinkel, St. Jude trustees found precisely the combination of talents they had been looking for in their first hospital director.

"Moving from Roswell Park Memorial Cencer Institute in Buffalo to head up St. Jude was kind of a chance phenomenon. An old friend, Dr. Michael James Sweeney, told me about a group of well-to-do lay people in Southern California and Memphis, led by the entertainer Danny Thomas, who wanted to build a research hospital, but they were having difficulty locating a director because so few pediatricians in the United States were also working in leukemia.

"Jim Sweeney suggested I go look at the job. In the spring of 1961, I met with the search committee—physicians from the University of Tennessee College of Medicine and from the Memphis community—and was shown the new hospital under construction. It was sort of sitting off all by itself alongside a community hospital and about a mile away from the Medical School. I looked at it and thought, 'No way.'

"I was only thirty-four at the time, so my feeling was that this would be an interesting job for somebody else. But then I met some of the philanthropists behind this venture and was impressed with their sincerity and their integrity. We talked all day long and found that, although our backgrounds were very different, our ideas about the hospital were almost identical and our philosophies and the way we thought about life and people were remarkably harmonious.

"After that meeting I expressed an interest in the position, because I saw an opportunity to develop an institution different from any that had ever existed. It would be a place where pediatrics and its objectives—the welfare and advocacy of children—would not be in constant competition for recognition within some existing university hospital. It would devote two-thirds or three-fourths of its space and resources to research. Scientifically and medically, the hospital founders would leave everything totally up to me and to the staff I'd recruit. There were other reasons for taking the position. The hospital would be completely free to all children—no accounts receivable—and would accept all children with diseases under study regardless of race, religion, or socioeconomic status. In addition, it would be racially integrated in every way, the first racially integrated medical institution in the Memphis region.

"More than anything else I was impressed by the sincerity of these people and the fact that they had looked for a director unsuccessfully for a year and a half and they were really at the bottom of the barrel. I thought, 'Somebody has got to come along. Somebody has to do this.' And I said to my friends, 'It's a big chance. But I'm young enough that if I fall on my face I have time to get up again.' So I signed on in July of 1961. The major part of the hospital was completed by about February 1962, and we opened the doors for our patients on March 16, 1962.

"It was plenty scary. I walked in there in 1961 and saw this empty building, and it was up to me to set up everything."

Dr. Pinkel started to do laboratory work right away. He set up one room as a laboratory, hired a technician, and was growing tumor cells in tissue culture by the second week he was there. But his biggest immediate challenge was to get the clinical services going: inpatient ward, outpatient clinic, nursing unit, clinical laboratories, x-ray department, blood bank, and so forth.

The founding of the volunteer blood bank exemplified Don Pinkel's creative talents as an administrator. An effective blood bank is essential to the care of leukemic children. Memphis had two commercial blood banks, financially tied to the pathologists in town. These blood banks were buying blood from donors off the street for $5 a unit and selling it to the hospitals for about $15 a unit, and the hospitals were charging the patient about $35 a unit. St. Jude could have gone broke very quickly buying blood from this market.

"I broke the blood banks, you might say, by beginning a volunteer donor system in Memphis." Don began by asking his new acquaintances in town who might be willing to give blood for free. One friend of the hospital put Don in touch with an admiral and a marine colonel at Millington Naval Air Station; sailors and marines there were volunteering to give blood. Don also recruited Memphis college students and fraternal groups as blood donors.

Then the warden of the nearby penal farm visited the hospital, was shown the children in the leukemia ward, and asked his inmates to help. The prisoners were happy to have the opportunity to get off the penal farm, and they got a good dinner in return. They also derived a good deal of satisfaction from doing something so worthwhile.

To fill other needs of the new hospital, Don again took the direct approach. "Our children with cancer needed dental care—infected teeth and gums can be a source of fatal bacteremia as well as much discomfort. Most dentists were understandably reluctant to treat these children in their offices. So I went looking around Washington for support for a dentist and a dental clinic, and after two days discovered a sympathetic ear in the Bureau of State Services of the Department of Health, Education and Welfare (HEW). This bright and personable dentist/administrator visited St. Jude and looked at the mouths of my children with leukemia, cried a little, and sat down and worked out a plan for us to receive support from his bureau. Some years later I received a phone call from HEW telling me that this man had died suddenly and that his fellow employees wished to send contributions to St. Jude in his memory. They felt that this was what he would wish most. Sometimes one hears about 'impersonal federal bureaucracy,' but I always found warm, sensitive persons in every HEW office.

"At St. Jude we provided free drugs, transportation, and room and board to our patients as well as free medical and hospital care. With the high price of anticancer drugs and some antibiotics, our pharmacy costs were potentially very high. What saved us in the early years was the fantastic generosity of several pharmaceutical manufacturers, who filled our orders without billing us, and the National Cancer Institute, which sent us most of the anticancer drugs from its stocks.

"The leaders of the National Cancer Institute were also a tremendous help to us when it came to our biggest challenge: recruiting staff of high quality even though we didn't have much money. In the early years Doctors Ken Endicott and Palmer Saunders came down from NCI for three days and saw what we were trying to do. They were really helpful in promoting St. Jude as a children's cancer center. I wonder whether they could do such a thing today, with so many different levels of approval required. One reason these people were interested in helping us get started was that there was no other cancer center in the South then, and there was criticism that all of the cancer research money was going to other parts of the country. But mostly the NCI officials wanted to help children with cancer, and St. Jude was the best way.

"Throughout, we continued to have a very good relationship with the lay people who began this venture. The main fund raiser, American-Lebanese-Syrian Associated Charities, continued its support and enthusiasm. Danny Thomas was involved in all of this and used to say, 'This country has been very good to us as Lebanese and Syrian Americans. We are very grateful for the hospitality of this country and we want to show this country our gratitude and we want to give something back that's important.'

"Curiously we rarely got Lebanese or Syrian American patients, and there was never any pressure about bringing patients in from Lebanon or excluding any group of people. The lay leadership never tried to second-guess us. They just gave as a complete gift from the heart and were very energetic, hard-working, committed people.

"But the expenses were very great. It reached the point where about half of the income was from money raised privately and half was grants from the National Cancer Institute, the American Cancer Society, and other agencies. Altogether we had a strong combination of supporting groups. That was the important underpinning for our scientific investigations.

''We were only open for about three months when, in the summer of 1962, we began wondering if we could *cure* leukemia rather than just treat it to gain temporary remission. There were a lot of concepts being talked about in 1962. We had the benefit of new information: that combination chemotherapy seemed to be more effective than chemotherapy with single drugs, and that certain drugs were superior for producing remission whereas other drugs were better for continuing remission. We knew from the work of Howard Skipper, Abe Goldin, Frank Schabel, and others that L_{1210} mouse leukemia could be cured. But we also knew that something had to be done for our children who experienced central nervous system (CNS) relapse, that is, relapse occurring in the covering of the brain and spinal cord. Giving drugs by mouth or by vein was simply not enough to offset the problem of relapse in the CNS region. So we developed a plan.

"First we would produce a remission by the use of steroids and vincristine in order to get the patient out of the woods. We had to convert what looked like a terminally ill patient into one who seemed to have at most an early stage of leukemia. Then we had the notion that, when the child had recovered sufficient strength and was producing normal blood cells, we would add an intensive phase of chemotherapy in order to reduce the leukemia cell population much more. After that, we would use long-term chemotherapy with those drugs that were most useful for prolonging the remission. Our thought was that some leukemias would be sensitive to all of the drugs that we used, and we might be able to cure that group. But we knew that there was a blood/spinal fluid barrier that made it inefficient to get certain drugs into the CNS. So another idea was to give radiation treatment to the CNS as a way of killing off leukemic cells without depending upon drugs going from the bloodstream into the spinal fluid.

"In the summer of 1962 we started out with the first study of what we called 'total therapy,' and we went from there. Five years later we'd reached the point where it was clear that the use of multiple drug combination chemotherapy resulted in more frequent and longer remissions than we'd ever seen before, but our method of preventing leukemia in the CNS was still unsatisfactory; half of the children with acute leukemia were still experiencing initial relapse in the CNS. However, we had also innovated by stopping therapy after two or three years of continuous complete remission. We now had the experience of having taken seven youngsters off treatment in 1966—and all were still in remission in 1967. So we thought that it looked as though curing childhood acute leukemia *was* possible, because we'd had some of our children who had been intensively treated and who were now off therapy and staying in remission and showing no risk of relapse.

"Stopping therapy was a momentous decision to make, because at that time to stop chemotherapy could have meant death for the children when their leukemia recurred. Yet if the patient had been finally cured, then the additional unnecessary treatments might cause harmful long-term effects. But no one was anxious to quit treatment while this child was doing well. So it was hard, really hard, to stop treatment initially. But we knew by 1967 that seven children had been off therapy for a year, and they were still well. There was a curious thing that happened that we had to learn about because, after all, this was uncharted territory. There were no guidelines or experts to consult. We found that some of the children who had been taken off therapy for only a short time developed abnormal-looking cells in their marrow after the treatment was stopped, and it looked at first like a recurrence of the leukemia. That was scary! What it was, though, was a 'pseudo-relapse,' which means that for a period of time immature or young, normal cells were appearing in the bone marrow. After we had stopped the drugs, these cells appeared in the marrow—but they were *not* leukemic cells even though they had a superficial resemblance to leukemic cells. In fact, it was very difficult with the tools we had at that time to tell the difference, and it was frightening until we learned that it was a normal phenomenon of recovery from chemotherapy effects. That was a relief.

"But despite some of this initial success, we were discouraged that about 85 percent of our children were still dying of leukemia. CNS relapse was the initial relapse site in the majority, so we decided that we'd make another experimental attempt to prevent this complication. We knew by then that giving methotrexate into the spinal fluid did not produce a very high drug concentration in the brain area, and so we needed to give sufficient radiation to the brain itself to supplement the drug. We increased the dosage of cranial radiation to 2,400 rads—double what we'd ever given before. We confined the radiation to the head. We were concerned about the effects of radiation on bone growth in the spine; we didn't want to arrest the growth of the child. So instead of radiating the spinal column, we used methotrexate injected into the spinal fluid in order to bathe the spinal meninges with this leukemia-killing drug.

"Our chemotherapy plan was to continue using steroids and vincristine to produce a remission and then give a week of intravenous 6-MP, methotrexate, and cyclophosphamide in order to solidify the remission. Then we'd go on with what we call continuation therapy for about two years using oral and intravenous medication, including 6-MP, methotrexate, and cyclophosphamide.

"We saw a difference almost right away! The relapse rate in the CNS was less, and the overall relapse rate was also less. Actually thirty-one of thirty-five consecutive children with acute lymphoid leukemia went into remission, and nineteen of these children are still in remission today, more than twenty-five years later. That was the first time anyone had established a 50 percent continuous remission rate, free of all further treatment. We began that study in December of 1967, and by June it was obvious that these children were going to do better. At that point I said, 'OK, we must do a comparative study to learn whether it's the treatment that we're giving to the nervous system or the different *way* in which we're giving our chemotherapy that is reducing the CNS relapse rate.'

"The comparative study forced parents of leukemic children at St. Jude into making terrifying decisions. They knew that the disease was fatal without treatment. They knew that the standard treatments could only stave off relapse, not prevent it—except for that tiny hopeful minority who had been off treatment for more than a year and were still in remission. They were told that the experimental treatments of high doses of radiation were potentially very dangerous. And if they agreed to put their child in the study, they had no choice in the treatment: the patients in the study were assigned randomly to one treatment or the other." Would *you* volunteer your five-year-old for a new treatment program that might kill the child even more rapidly than the leukemia in the hope of a favorable response, just possibly even a cure? In his long discussions with parents, Don Pinkel could draw on his experience early in his career when, as a pediatric resident, he had had to advise parents of children with congenital heart defects.

"In the early 1950s they were just beginning to do surgery for congenital heart disease in children. Surgeons had perfected the operation of tying off the patent ductus, a blood vessel abnormality that could result in serious infection later on. However, they were just beginning to do more complicated heart surgery to repair other heart defects. The death rate from surgery alone was about 50 percent for some of these procedures. One of our jobs as residents was to sit down, along with the attending cardiologist, with the family and explain that if we did not do the surgery, the youngster might live another year but eventually would die of irreversible heart failure, and that with surgery there might be a mortality of 50 percent at the time of operation, but that if the child survived the surgery there might be a much longer survival and much better quality of life. That was a very difficult dilemma for parents. We got somewhat accustomed to presenting this choice, as heart-wrenching as it was. Parents often chose the risk of immediate surgical death over the certainty of slow death. As time went on and the surgical techniques improved, more and more children survived.

"Now in the area of leukemia we were doing experimental treatments in children with the knowledge that untreated children would all die within a year, as would children treated conventionally with single drugs, so the decision wasn't quite that difficult. Furthermore, the treatments that we used were not so toxic for the most part. True, there would be an increased risk of infection and bleeding and serious complications, but there wasn't the great risk that we would kill patients, at least not with those early chemotherapy programs. One argument that was used against our program of combination chemotherapy—the argument that I heard more than any other—was that if you used up all the drugs at one time, what would you do when the patient relapsed from that treatment? But I found, in discussing this with families and weighing the possibility of a longer life, that they could understand that process. We did mention the possibility that we were trying to achieve a long remission—I never used the word cure— and we thought we might be able to do that if we used combination chemotherapy even though it would add risks to the patient. The parents recognized that we would also have to face the fact that if the child relapsed, then there was virtually nothing left. When we went through this type of fairly complicated explanation, they were almost uniformly willing to accept those risks.

"The emotional and psychological impact was the same, no matter what the educational level of the parents. In fact leukemia, or cancer in general, is a great leveler. The very educated and highly sophisticated and those who are not sophisticated or well educated come to a common plane, because it's something you have to deal with emotionally and not rationally.

"These sorts of things tear you up inside, and your family and friends can't understand what's happening at times. Yet I'd rather face these problems and make progress for the children than not move ahead. We are constantly learning, and that can make it better for the next patient, possibly even a matter of life and death. It was a great satisfaction to find, thanks to this comparative study and others that followed it, that the powerful radiation treatments were indeed bringing about many more cures."

Don Pinkel is optimistic that eventually we will be able to cure virtually 100 percent of children with leukemia. "Well, I'm not sure *when* we will get there, but we're certainly closer than we were five or ten years ago. It is my belief that as we learn more about the genetics of leukemia and as we begin to target our chemotherapy more accurately in relationship to the genetic abnormalities in leukemia, that we will have more precise and effective treatment. We have a lot of investigation to do in this regard, but I think I see a way to do it now—and it's going to make a big difference. There is no question that the future lies in the development of even better chemotherapy, and of course we're now able to cure a very large fraction of children by the use of chemotherapy. We just need more refined ways of using the drugs, and we need more and better drugs. Where are the new drugs going to come from? I think these drugs are going to come from industry, and the pharmaceutical industry is tooling up to do more and better research. They're getting highly qualified people and building additional facilities. I do believe that the United States has lost a good deal of its leadership in chemotherapy partly because of the Food and Drug Administration—the FDA has been choking us all.

"As we learn more about the details of leukemia at the genetic level, which is where it's happening, I believe, we'll be able to treat all of the children more effectively. The eventual solution to the problem of childhood leukemia is prevention. We need vigorous renewal of efforts to identify causation and prevention of leukemia utilizing the rapidly expanding information and technology of molecular genetics. In the meantime we should be more concerned about simplifying leukemia therapy and making curative treatment more available and accessible to all children in need."

PART V

The Lucky Ones

In the early days of leukemia research in the 1950s and 1960s, virtually all the children in the studies died. However, one thing was sure—if a child had acute leukemia and *wasn't* able to be in such a program, the outcome was bound to be fatal. The patients who participated in the studies were trailblazers, whether they made it or not. All future survivors of this disease owe them a debt of gratitude.

But what was it like for those lucky few who made it? How did they feel about the treatments they both needed and feared? How did they and their families cope? And how did their experience with leukemia affect their lives afterwards?

Now it is time to hear the words of some of the survivors, the children—now grown up—and adults whose lives testify to the success of the research chronicled here. In occasional instances the names are changed. The dates when their illnesses were first diagnosed span almost a quarter of a century, from 1954 to 1977, and their survival illustrates not only the cure of acute lymphocytic leukemia but also the vanquishing of other kinds of cancer by the principles of treatment learned from childhood leukemia research.

Debbie Brown

Every once in a while, one of Dr. Joseph Burchenal's patients at Memorial Sloan-Kettering had a startlingly lengthy remission, but it took a long time for anyone to think that the child might in fact have been cured. Debbie Brown, first diagnosed with leukemia in 1954, may well be the first and longest-term survivor on Joe's books. Today she lives with her husband and daughter in New Jersey.

I got leukemia in the summer of 1954, when I was nine, going into third grade; but I really didn't know I had it until I was about fifteen or sixteen. I was very very tired. We lived on the second floor, and I had to crawl up the stairs because I was so tired. All I wanted to do was sleep. I bruised very easily. My parents were in the process of getting a divorce the same month I got sick. The leukemia was an additional strain, especially for my mother. (My brother, who is six years younger than I, and I lived with our mother, but I stayed very close to my father.)

My parents took me to the doctor. I was told later on that Dr. Arvalla thought it was leukemia and first put me in the local hospital, where they did blood tests and bone marrow tests. Dr. Arvalla wanted a definite diagnosis; he knew about Memorial Sloan-Kettering, and he told my parents to take me there. I was mostly an outpatient and only stayed in the hospital as an inpatient a couple of times. First I saw Dr. Burchenal—he's a sweetheart—and he referred me to Dr. Lois Murphy and Dr. Charlotte Tan. In the beginning I went in about three times a week.

At first they gave me a new 6-MP and another drug called azaserine together; later they put me on methotrexate. I was supposed to take it constantly, but the methotrexate would give me a rash in my mouth. So I'd go off the drug for a while; then, when the rash cleared up a little, I'd go back on the medicine again. I had to keep a chart of when I had the rash and when I took the medicine.

I took myself off the medicine. I figured that, well, if I could be without it for a week or two and I was fine—I was going back periodically for testing and they kept showing I was fine—then why take it? [Note: This is not a good way to take such potent medicine, although it apparently did no harm in this instance.]

When I first got the disease, I was really sick. I couldn't go to school, and the school system paid for a tutor for about three years. It didn't bother me at first, but as I felt better, I was a little rebellious. I don't think my mother was too happy that I was going back to school, because she was still trying to be protective. But when I finally felt good, I didn't see any reason not to go to high school.

When I was in high school I overheard my mother talking to someone and that was how I learned I had leukemia. My mother came from the old-fashioned school where you don't tell children things, because you're afraid they'll be upset. So she was reluctant to say I had it even then. Finally, after I got enough facts together, I confronted her with it, and she did admit that I had leukemia. She still doesn't like to talk about my illness, although my father and I talk about it sometimes.

I had seen very very sick kids with leukemia in the hospital. I remember how they had lost their hair and I remember that, when I came back the next time, they weren't there anymore. But the doctors really played that down and didn't come right out and say they had died.

By the point I finally learned I had leukemia, though, the knowledge didn't really bother me. By then I wasn't sick anymore. I was only going into the hospital about once a month for a check-up. I wasn't taking the medicine anymore. I was going to school and functioning like a normal person.

After high school I went to nursing school for a year and a half. I'd always liked hospital work and to be around people, helping them. (I'm not sure if that's from my earlier days in the hospital or what—the people at Memorial had really treated us pretty nicely.)

Then I got married. After we'd been dating awhile, I told my husband-to-be about the leukemia. It didn't seem to bother him, because at that point I was considered cured, although Dr. Burchenal never really came out and said I was cured—it was almost like an understanding after I'd gone so many years without the disease coming back. I had a perfectly normal pregnancy—the doctors said there didn't seem to be any reason why we shouldn't have children—and our daughter was born in 1969. Now I am a teacher.

Looking back on it all, I just think I was blessed and very lucky. It was an experience that makes you stronger as a person and appreciate life. You have more compassion for people who have problems in their lives, because you've gone through something in your own life that makes you try to understand them better.

James Eversull

James Eversull was diagnosed as having acute lymphocytic leukemia in 1964. On November 17, 1966, he was taken off all therapy, the first child to reach that important milestone at St. Jude. Today James is a normal adult, working in Lafayette, Louisiana.

—*1987 St. Jude Silver Anniversary Report*

My parents were the first to receive the devastating news: "Your son has leukemia." Being only one and a half years old when I began my visits to St. Jude Children's Research Hospital, I can't recall my early days and only know what I was told. However, I made regular visits to the hospital for eighteen years, until I was one of the lucky ones considered to be cured. I remember the other children there, hooked up to intravenous bottles, screaming, whining, and getting shots. And I also remember myself having bone marrow samples taken and getting shots. I didn't like the shots, but kept getting them anyway. I didn't like the bone marrow tests either, but I wouldn't cry and that shocked people. I would just grit my teeth and keep on going. They'd have to wrap me in a sheet, and there would be about three doctors to hold me while the doctor did the bone marrow or spinal tap. Still I remember that everyone was friendly and nice and went out of their way to help in any way they could. Over the course of the years I went through three or four different doctors. I started out with one and he ended up moving or getting another job offer in another place, and I would go to another doctor, and another, and another, so I really didn't settle with any one.

They gave me pills and medicine to try to help me. Some of the pills tasted like oranges so I chewed a whole bunch of them and had to go to the doctor for an overdose. All told, I only had to have chemotherapy for about a year or so, but then I had to go back for about eight years of follow-up to get the bone marrow tests done. Still, when I was about nine or ten years old, I didn't want anyone to know that I had leukemia because I'd

244

seen television programs where the other kids would treat you like, "Get away from me, you're not like me, you've got a disease, you're going to give it to me." By that time I was over the chemotherapy and the lumbar puncture treatments and the radiation to the brain, and I looked and acted pretty normal. I was really tickled when the doctors told me that I didn't have to get the bone marrow tests anymore, although they also told me that I had to keep coming back, at first every two years, and then they moved it up to every four years, and finally they put me on "alumni status" because I was cured.

I was excited and happy on that day because I was one of the first of the original patients that was cured. The doctors said they really didn't have an idea of what they had done to cure me. They said they couldn't explain it—they said it was like some kind of miracle. And then when I would go back periodically, I'd just go around and talk to some of the parents there who looked like they were upset, and they would even let me visit some of the kids who were in the hospital. I had a chance to tell them that there was a good opportunity for them to be cured, but I would feel sad when I would go in to see a very sick child, and I'd start having memories of my looking like that. But I'd walk in and try to look cheerful and not let it bother me that they didn't have hair and were vomiting from their chemotherapy or whatever. I'd sit down and talk with the children, and some of them were crying. I even cried with one girl; her parents felt that she didn't have a chance, and she was getting weaker and weaker. I tried telling the parents that if they would try to keep up their spirits and keep up their attitude and help her fight for her life, you know, try to keep going, that she'd have a chance. And they ended up going back to see the girl and telling her, "You see that guy, he had what you have, and he's still alive and walking around and he's considered cured." The girl ended up smiling and that made me feel as though I'd accomplished something, and if she didn't make it, at least I know she smiled once more. I was about sixteen then.

Unfortunately, that girl didn't make it. She died, and I got a nice letter from one of her parents. I cried a little and was upset, because I thought that if she would fight for her life she would make it, like me. I wanted every one of them to make it, and if it were up to me, they all would have made it.

All together, I visited about ten children after being cured, and all of them made it except three. It made me feel good that those seven children had made it, and perhaps something I had told them and my seeing them made them feel better and helped them to fight for life, to keep going, to have hope to continue on with the treatments.

It was a tough thing for my parents and my grandmother, all of whom would go with me to St. Jude every time I'd have to make a visit. We'd fly or something, according to what we could afford. Fortunately, the program at the hospital paid for the treatments. I had a lot of fine doctors and Dr. Pinkel was one of them, Dr. Green was another, and I don't remember all the names. But none of the old people are there now and when I go back to visit it seems kind of weird, because there's nobody left for me to talk to who knew me from those days.

One of my early recollections has to do with needles. I was so scared of needles, particularly the long one for the spinal tap, and I'd always yell and kick and everything. Then I'd see all the other kids crying and hollering and how people were trying to keep them steady, and I said, "Well, I don't want them to have that problem with me," and so I'd sit there and grit my teeth and let them hold me and go about and do it.

When this was all done with, I continued my schooling. I made A's, B's and C's, and nothing below a C. After two years in college studying business administration, I had to quit school and work to make some money because the expenses at school kept going up. Right now I'm working as a contractor, repairing gas lines here in the Lafayette, Louisiana, area. We look for gas leaks and if we find one in the gas line, then we dig it up and repair it.

I've been doing some volunteer coaching for the last seven years in basketball and girls' softball, and now I think I'd like to be a coach. In my own youth, I was able to get on the wrestling team and the football team, and I tried very hard to live a normal life. I do feel like a normal person, and don't even think about my leukemia anymore, except when someone brings it up and starts talking about leukemia or cancer, and then I sort of freeze. I don't really want to touch on the subject. But I am proud to be living a normal life, and I have a girlfriend and a normal social life.

At first I thought I would not be able to have children because of the chemotherapy, but I've been tested for that and I am able to have children. So that's one thing I'd been scared about.

I was lucky to have my parents and my grandmother there with me when I was going through this illness. I have a brother and a sister, but I couldn't really talk to them about my pain. I don't think anybody could really understand the pain you went through and all the suffering and sadness that was going on around you. Maybe they could, but I wish people wouldn't feel the way they do when they find out that you have a disease. Then they just sort of panic, they tend to treat you differently—like you're more fragile and you can't do this or that. And that's the way my parents were at first. But then we'd go to visit the pediatrician, and the doctors would say, "Let him lead a normal life, let him do what he wants to do." Finally my parents slacked off and let me do what I wanted, and when I showed that I could handle the sports, then they said, "OK, he can do it, let him do it."

There's one way in which I think I'm different today than if I hadn't had my illness. I live every day like it's going to be my last day. My philosophy is to live life to the fullest and enjoy yourself, because I think that somebody helped me. I don't know if it was me and the doctors or maybe Him upstairs who helped me out. But I know that on more than one occasion, the doctors pretty much gave up on me and somehow I made it through. One time a priest came in and said the last rites for me, but by the next morning I had improved, and I felt that He had some reason for having saved me. He wanted me to survive in the world. I do love working with people, and I love people altogether and I try to help them. I feel sad for anybody that's disabled and handicapped, and I'm always trying to help them if I can in any way.

Charlotte Boozer
and Her Parents

In 1975, Charlotte Boozer was found to have acute promyelocytic leukemia. She was eight years old. Today, Charlotte is a college student at Carson-Newman College in Jefferson City, Tennessee, where she is studying to become an elementary school teacher.

Charlotte

Sometimes when I'm driving my car or walking down a crowded street I look around at all the people I see and think to myself, "Why me? Why did it have to happen to me?" Out of all the people passing by I wonder how many have had a life-threatening illness. I come up with almost zero.

If I could go back and live my life over again I wouldn't change a thing—not even my experience with acute promyelocytic leukemia. That may sound strange, but as I wonder "Why me," I realize that I wouldn't, for anything in the world, trade the experience of having fought a serious fight and won.

Above all things I cherish is the fact that because of my sickness I became a stronger person, a fighter. Being so small, at age eight, and so weak through the ordeal, and having to fight off such a "big" disease, has made me realize that I can overcome any obstacle that life might throw at me. I really believe that it was in God's plan for me. And the most important part of fighting cancer and other catastrophic illness is believing. I mean *really* believing—keeping one's faith strong and holding it close to the heart.

I am so fortunate to have a family who loves and cares for me very much, and who was and is always there when I need them. I would not have made it had it not been for their prayers and presence, and those of friends. And of course, God and St. Jude Hospital.

To sum it up in one word, I think I'd say "precious." Precious because it was such a unique experience, overcoming such odds and growing up, making it through grade school, high school, and now college. It is something that will be forever with me, that I'll never forget. And precious because life is so precious.

It is such a shame that it takes almost dying to realize the gift we've all been given in just being alive. Now it doesn't seem as if it ever happened. I see pictures of a very sick and skinny bald little girl and can hardly believe my eyes. There is so much about the illness that I cannot recall because I blocked it out of my mind, and the things I don't remember are probably the things that frightened me most. What I do remember is what matters the most. I remember the love and prayers of everyone around me, the feeling of being considered something special. Above all, I remember the feeling of God being everywhere around me and my family. That is what I'll never forget—the things that love and faith can do.

Mrs. Carol Boozer, Mother

We had just moved from Memphis to Nashville, and Charlotte had just had her eighth birthday party. We were planning to go back to Memphis to attend the wedding of her piano teacher and one morning, just before we left, I noticed blood on her pillow. I checked her mouth and didn't see anything wrong, but I made an appointment to see our pediatrician back in Memphis. When we got down there he looked at Charlotte and said, "Well, I don't know what I'm looking at, but I don't like what I see. I want you to go to the hospital in the morning to have some blood tests done." I asked him if I should be worried and he said, "Don't worry until I tell you to," and I tried hard not to worry. The next morning we went in to have the tests, and the doctor at LeBonheur Children's Hospital said that he wanted some other doctors from St. Jude Children's Research Hospital to come over and check Charlotte, and I knew immediately that it was something serious. They came over, examined her, did a bone marrow test, and then they took us over to St. Jude Hospital. They told me briefly what they thought the problem was and asked me to sign some papers. This was probably the hardest thing I'd ever done in my life, to sign my child away!

I frankly don't remember what was in the papers, but they had to do with the fact that she would be treated with experimental drugs. I was in a state of shock at the time, but I talked with my wonderful pediatrician and he said that this was the best thing that could be done for her. My husband was still back in Nashville, so I signed the papers and they took Charlotte upstairs and put her in a germ-free isolation room, which had air circulating through it all the time to keep it germ-free. And I was in the room adjacent to it with a glass wall between Charlotte and myself. It was pretty traumatic.

The doctors told me, "Sometimes patients don't make it through the first twenty-four hours—the initial shock of the chemotherapy kills them." I had to call my husband in Nashville and ask him to come to the hospital. I told him the doctor said it was pretty serious, but I didn't dare tell him that she might not live for another day because I didn't want him driving for two hundred miles with that knowledge. Dr. Joseph V. Simone of St. Jude was just wonderful to Charlotte, and anyway, she wasn't old enough to really be scared. The boy in the next room was sixteen and he was scared to death, but Charlotte was not. When Dr. Simone went in to talk to Charlotte, he told her, "You have a disease. It's like a field where you're trying to grow flowers and the weeds keep coming up, and we have to try to get rid of the weeds and grow more flowers." Charlotte understood that.

It was three months before she went into a remission, and when she did and Dr. Simone told her the good news, she said, "Does that mean my weeds are all gone?" So that really made an impression on her.

For the first ten days she received intensive treatment, and then we were on once a week treatments until she was in remission, and after that we came back every other week for three months. And we killed a couple of cars driving back and forth between Nashville and Memphis, a round trip of four hundred miles.

I'm a very firm believer in the importance of attitude in how you respond to your treatment, even though there's nothing scientific about that. But I feel that if the parents have a very positive attitude that it's going to help the child so much, and I tried very hard to make the trips down there fun for Charlotte. We'd go right after school, and we'd always go and get one of her friends and then go out to dinner, go skating, do anything to have a good time. Then we'd go to the hospital at 8:00 the next morning, and she would throw up just as soon as we drove into the parking lot. The doctors call that anticipatory vomiting, a conditioned response to having had vomiting after chemotherapy. She associated that parking lot with the chemotherapy, and that was enough to make her vomit. Charlotte couldn't understand why the medicines had to make her vomit if they were supposed to make her feel better. But we had had fun the night before each visit, and while we were there at the hospital, after the check-ups, while we were waiting for the medicine we always had an hour or two, and we'd go somewhere

250

to eat—we didn't eat there in the hospital. She was able to eat, although then she'd throw it up—but nevertheless she would try. And she continued to have trouble with vomiting as long as she was receiving chemotherapy.

Charlotte was on chemotherapy for a total of thirty months. The children who had gone to school with her in the third grade and on up knew about her leukemia, and it was OK for them to know, but she didn't want anyone else to know about it. When she was in high school, she certainly didn't want anybody to know. And I thought that that was so sad, because she is a miracle child. In her senior year in high school she did come around by herself. She wrote a paper that was submitted to one of the magazines for a contest, in which she described her experience, and that kind of broke the ice for her. It didn't win a prize, but since that time she's been more open about it. Now she's in college and willing to share her experience and, in fact, has written some other articles. We are members of the Baptist church, and she's written some pieces for Baptist magazines. That makes sense to her because she realizes that it was a miracle that her life was saved, and she's willing to share that knowledge.

Charlotte had something called acute promyelocytic leukemia, and Dr. Simone told us that the chances of a cure might only be less than 1 percent, and that there had been no one who had ever been cured of it prior to that time. When the doctor told us that she might have eight to ten months or a year to live if we were lucky, I really thought this was the beginning of the end. I thought I was prepared to handle it. But I wasn't as prepared as I thought I was. When I got to the hospital one time, I had to carry her in from the car because she was too weak to walk and she was hemorrhaging from everyplace—her mouth, her ears, her nose, and everything. After the doctors took her, I went to the phone and called my minister in Memphis and said, "Could you please come down here and stay with me?"

Here we are, twelve years later, and she's a healthy young woman, and as of last year, she doesn't go for annual check-ups anymore. She's had her last visit and received a formal release. Any future trips will be for "alumni" gatherings of former patients. One of the big blessings has been that she wasn't physically or emotionally changed, either by the disease or by the treatments. She's grown up and she's a beautiful young woman. She has a 3.7 average at college and is an honor student, running cross-country track in the mountains of East Tennessee. We see a miracle every time we look at her.

Mr. William Boozer, Father

Curiously, there are parts of Charlotte's experience with leukemia that she doesn't remember having gone through. When I first learned about Charlotte's illness, it was devastating for me. I had been working as a writer for a newspaper in Memphis and had recently joined the Memphis Chamber of Commerce when Danny Thomas came to town in the early stages of planning for St. Jude, and so I was familiar with St. Jude and the kind of work that they did, and of course Carol was too. The roof fell in on us because both of us knew the kind of cases that they handled—catastrophic diseases. So when I got a call at 3:00 P.M. on October 11, 1975, I got in the car and drove to Memphis in record time. I only recall that my mind was racing back to 1960, when Danny Thomas was attempting to get St. Jude going, and here I was, heading there.

It was tough on all of us. We have two older boys (now in their twenties) as well, and we tried not to deprive them of attention because of Charlotte's illness. Our friends and neighbors were very good to them, and the illness didn't seem to affect their lives too much. The closest we may have come to seeing something break was when Charlotte's platelets had gone to zero. The doctors said they were going to put Charlotte back in the hospital, and Carol announced to Bart and Brandon that she was going to have to take Charlotte back to Memphis again, the third trip in four days. Bart, then thirteen years old, was on the verge of tears. Carol told me later that she was so exhausted that, if anybody had said anything, she wouldn't have been able to drive back. Charlotte was like a rag at that time, her platelet count was zero, her hemoglobin was extremely low, and our oldest child said, "Are you going to have to go back to Memphis *again?*" And Carol said, "Yes, honey, Charlotte's not well and we're going to have to go back again." And he put his hand on his hip and told her, "I'm so tired of washing dishes!" Everybody needed that laugh!

Clay Johnson

Think about being a young child suddenly stricken with an illness that renders you powerless and afraid. You count on your parents to nurture you and make you well. But suppose they have to send you far away from home to get painful treatments, and suppose they too feel powerless. How do you survive? Children are remarkably resilient, and Clay, for one, not only survived the experience but has interesting recollections that have shaped his life.

The diagnosis of leukemia wasn't made correctly for a long time, and apparently that isn't uncommon. Our home was in Peoria in 1977, and I was eight years old. We were on a vacation in Florida, when my temperature went up to 104 degrees, and I had pain in my joints, swollen joints and a rash. It was right around Christmas time, and I was really sick. My parents picked this doctor out of the Yellow Pages of the phone book at this vacation resort. Apparently acute leukemia commonly resembles juvenile rheumatoid arthritis, and it had seemed to my doctor that I was a textbook case, with arthritis, fever, rash, and everything. So he treated me with high doses of aspirin, which I later learned isn't particularly good for patients with leukemia (it increases the tendency to bleed), and he sent me home. However, I tolerated the aspirin for three and a half months, and we varied the dose according to how bad the pain was in my joints. But when my blood count began to drop, with the hemoglobin falling to 5, my pediatrician said, "Hey, something's up," and I had my first bone marrow test. That was in April of 1978, and it was done by a pathologist in Peoria who told me briefly what I really had, but didn't explain it to me clearly. I was immediately referred to St. Jude and we arrived in Memphis shortly afterwards.

I'd never heard of St. Jude or of Memphis, but when we were told to go there, we must have left Peoria around 6:00 at night and got there at 2:00 in the morning. We went right in, and they said, "Come back tomorrow." That's when they diagnosed it, after the initial bone marrow, and the final tests were done the next morning, on April 24. And so it was kind of a strange road to the diagnosis of acute lymphocytic leukemia.

Dr. Gary Dahl told me immediately after the first bone marrow test at St. Jude that I had leukemia, and he explained to me, in simple lay terms, what that meant, what was going on in my body and what they would do about it. Of course, I wasn't feeling too much about anything at the time because I was so sick, and I had 50 percent leukemic blast cells in my blood and a high fever and just plain felt sick. I was drifting in and out of a restless sleep and really wasn't thinking about much of anything except the next few minutes.

My parents were really scared. The tension was obvious in both my mom and my dad, and Dad always looked really serious. It was clear to me that they were trying not to make it obvious that they were scared, if you know what I mean. They were also asking some serious "why" questions; but our family has always had a very strong faith in God. So there was an attitude of, "Well, if we have to have it, we'll let God take care of it," and the thing that brought me through is my knowledge that God would never give me anything that I couldn't handle, and if He did, well then I would be in Paradise. That's the one thought that really did bring me through, even as a young child.

There were a number of people at the hospital who were important to me. There were many doctors, but Gary Dahl was the main man. And Andi Wood, the nurse practitioner, at one point saved my life. Not long after the treatments began, my white count was close to zero, and I developed a little cut on the cuticle of my finger the very last day before we were scheduled to leave Memphis. Even though I cleaned the wound Andi said, "Just to be on the safe side, we'll culture it and see what happens." We returned to the hotel to pack. We were going to leave for Peoria around 9:00 the next morning. But around 6:30 or 7:00 in the morning, Andi called us and said that we should come in before we left. She'd been up all night worrying about that thing on my thumb and had simply waited for a decent time to call us. By that time my fever was 102 degrees, and I was bleeding into the skin. We rushed to the hospital. Had we left town, I think our station wagon would soon have become a hearse, because I went so quickly into septic shock. The doctors put me into the intensive care unit and gave me three kinds of antibiotics, which saved my life.

All in all, I wasn't in the hospital all that much. I was in the hospital for the first week and not much thereafter. Most of my treatment was as an outpatient, and I was cared for, in large part, by the Methodist Medical

Center in Peoria, which happens to be St. Jude's only affiliate. That was wonderful for me. But I would still work closely with the doctors from St. Jude, and my family would take me back periodically, though I was cared for at Methodist. I had radiation treatments to the brain (2,400 rads), plus regular chemotherapy, and chemotherapy in the spinal fluid: a lot of treatment. I went back to Memphis maybe once every three months for ten years after my disease became stabilized and I was in remission. It's a big trip from where we are, nine hours and 450 miles each way. Both my parents would accompany me, and we tried to make it a family outing. We'd never head back on the same day. For one thing, I learned that I had to stay flat on my back for a couple of hours after the spinal fluid examination and treatment; if I didn't, I would get a terrible headache, the worst that you can imagine.

This whole experience has brought our family closer together. In some ways it's given me a lot of opportunities I would never have had. If God would have come to me as an eight-year-old and said, "Look buddy, I'm going to give you leukemia, but you'll get all this out of it, and you'll still be alive in 1988"—I'd do it again. No one can understand that, but it's done such wonderful things for our family that it's worth all of the agony. I now have a sister thirty-two and a brother twenty-nine. My sister was very supportive of my illness, but my brother had trouble accepting it and relating to it. He had a middle child syndrome, and had a lot of his own problems, so he really couldn't face my illness. He was in college at the time and when I was the sickest, both he and my sister flew to Memphis to give me blood. That was a real sacrifice, because my brother faints at the sight of a needle. I ended up not needing the blood, though, so it turned out better than they thought it would. However, for one period of time I remember the doctor turning and saying to my father, "I'm so sorry." That had a certain meaning for Dad—he's a lawyer but he's also the son of an undertaker, and the phrase "I'm so sorry" has a very special connotation for undertakers. After all of this, my brother disappeared for fourteen months, his way of handling the scary situation.

Thanks to God, it never entered my mind that I was going to die. Somehow I just knew I was going to make it through, no matter what. But I wasn't naive about the situation, because during the time that I was in treatment, I even went to five or six funerals. These were for my friends who had leukemia and who died. When I was in grade school I had a lot of personal trouble dealing with my illness as well as trying to make it in the world of normal people. In fact, I lived more in a world of adults than children. My peers, my friends, were the people who were in the same predicament as I was. My friends were my acquaintances among these children with leukemia. It pained me deeply when they died. We went to a number of funerals and my parents accompanied me. They didn't try to talk me out of going to the funerals—in fact they urged me to go—but they were very sad and we all cried.

After I was cured we would still go back to St. Jude once a year, but my last visit to that hospital was last year. I'll always be grateful to the doctors and nurses. The one thing that was amazing to me was that there were no problems that I experienced that they couldn't understand. They always seemed to understand everything, and they went to the nth degree to solve the problem or at least listen, and even to try to cater to my wishes, which were sometimes unreasonable.

One time I had to be hospitalized on the unit for three weeks and I objected to the food, which was terrible—that was the only thing that was bad there. I actually went on a three-day hunger strike. There was one nurse who made me eat my hot food before I could get at the cold cereal, which was the only thing I liked, and I hated the whole thing. I was on prednisone at the time, and that gives you a ravenous appetite like you wouldn't believe—some children would rummage through the garbage can looking for food. At one point, I developed a craving for McDonald's fish sandwiches. So I went to Dr. Dahl, and he told me that they couldn't bring them to me because if one child had them, then everyone would want them. I was very upset at the time and very angry and the doctor walked out of the room and I threw a book at the door, and then he walked back into the room and he wasn't pleased with me. Well, there was another doctor there by the name of Dr. Rivira, who had once told me that if there was anything I ever needed to just give him a call. Imp that I was, I got on the phone and called Dr. Rivira, and I ended up getting my fish sandwich. It didn't seem to destroy the institution, but perhaps I shouldn't have done it anyway. But that was the only time I ever heard the word "no" in response to a request from me, and maybe that wasn't good for me either.

When I would go to the hospital, I didn't particularly dread the bone marrow and the spinal tap procedures, because I looked at it in the context that I was going to be down there for seventy-two hours or so, and that these two tests would take a maximum of four or five minutes, so I convinced myself that I should enjoy the whole experience. I always looked forward to going back. I really love the place, and managed the difficulties by being able to put the unpleasant things out of my mind. I don't know how I learned to do that as a way of handling problems. (The only problem for me now is that I can also do that with my schoolwork, and it's called daydreaming.) When I would have the bone marrow biopsies and spinal taps I would concentrate real hard on getting well, and I'd tell myself that it would be six months or whatever before I'd have to get another one.

I was aware that the treatment that I was getting was experimental and that the results were not guaranteed to work. Nobody survived in those days, but now there's better than a 50 percent survival rate. And so as things went on it became a lot less experimental, and I knew I was at the best place and never had any second thoughts about that at all. I'm really grateful to cancer research and leukemia research and to the people who support that, because that's the only way that we're going to be able to cure diseases in the future that are incurable today.

Some friends and I have worked very hard to raise money for research and have been fortunate to interest the teenagers in Peoria in a very success-ful fund-raising program. And that has been a very rewarding experience, even though it has been emotionally draining for me to discuss my personal experiences. You know, my age group is kind of hard to reach, and you can reach little old ladies a lot easier than you can sixteen- or seventeen-years-olds. First I told my story, and then we showed videotapes of a bone marrow and a spinal tap that were done on patients. Then we passed this huge spinal tap needle around and my friend Sherry told her story, and the audience really got involved. It was awfully hard for us, and they sensed that. If you can make them care, really deep down care, about the kid on the screen who's screaming his lungs out—and that's what happened. We recruited about a thousand kids from within the city limits. Then we had a fund-raiser and about 150 kids signed up to come to the kickoff dinner and that made me feel very good.

Another thing that is important for me to talk about is research on animals, because I feel that a whole lot of us wouldn't be alive without experimentation with animals. It's unfortunate that it's necessary, because I look on animals as creative beings just like us, but they aren't intelligent. It's a very sad thing to think about rats and monkeys and all other animals being kept in cages and used in research. Yet it's so important for what you get out of it—because of this research, some kid has a leg or a life, and that seems to justify using a large number of rats.

At the present time I'm studying at the University of Illinois at Urbana-Champaign, majoring in engineering. But I'm really a people person, and it's still possible that I might become a doctor. In some ways I've felt a compulsion to become a doctor or be otherwise associated with medicine. It's like feeling a responsibility to do this with my life. If I were to become a doctor, I'd be a pediatric oncologist, because it's a beautiful field. I've had a lot of medical problems and also trauma, being hit by a car, having a fractured skull as well as leukemia, and the way I look at it is that God has me alive for some reason. I'm still looking for that reason, where God will lead me, because by all rights I shouldn't be here. I think back on the days when I was having my chemotherapy and lost all my hair and having such a difficult time making it in the fourth grade because I had no friends, because I wasn't concerned about erasing the chalkboard for the teacher— I was concerned with living and dying. I had different priorities than my classmates, and I just didn't care about school. It was such a strain to be a bald, pale nine-year-old and have to change schools, as I did. But I made up my mind that I had to improve my attitude, and later, in high school, doors started opening up for me and it turned out to be great. Now I'm perhaps too much of a social creature, or so I hear. I enjoy dating and partying, and I'm not shy. I don't party too heavily because it's still a different life—I've still got twice the chance of developing cancer, and all of the possible complications that go with liver damage and everything—but I'm very lucky. I've been dating the same girl now for two years, and I don't foresee any reason why we won't be married someday, but that will be after our college educations.

[Some years later I received a letter from Clay. In it he told me that he had since graduated from the University of Illinois and had gone on to law school at Syracuse University. When he wrote, he was serving as a law clerk for a federal district judge in New York. He also commented further on his experience with leukemia.]

Regarding the war against leukemia, I am still in continuous complete remission and am currently struggling with the tension between putting the bad portions of the experience behind me and the complacency that such a desire can create. I am searching for a way to have the former without the latter. The experience is the primary basis for my personality, character, and attitudes and was overwhelmingly positive.

Were I to be given the choice of going through it before doing so and knowing the ultimate outcome, I would not hesitate to say yes. The short-term pain was worth the long-term benefits. (In my experience that is usually the case.) Of course, I am unable to say what I would choose were the outcome not revealed to me in advance, but it would be close.

Leslie Willig, Ph.D.

Les Willig wasn't a child and didn't have leukemia when he was treated by Dr. Frei. But he too was a pioneer because he had another kind of cancer that became curable as a consequence of research on childhood leukemia. Les is probably the first person ever cured of widespread Hodgkin's disease.

I first noticed a swelling above my left collar bone. When I showed it to my doctor, he looked at that and at my neck and wanted to take me right into the operating room for exploratory surgery. I was a little reluctant to go that route. At the time I knew nothing about Hodgkin's disease. So during the fall of 1966 the doctor did a number of blood tests, x-rays, and some other kinds of tests, and was unable to find any problem; he told me that I was in perfect health. I was forty at the time and physically in great shape. Finally, however, one of the x-rays showed a darkened area in the middle of my chest and as a result of that finding, he decided that I should have a biopsy of the nodes in the lower part of my neck on the left side. The biopsy determined that I had Hodgkin's disease. There were also some abnormal nodes under my left arm as well as in my chest, or mediastinum.

My doctors in Fort Wayne, Indiana, felt that mine was an early case, and they treated the areas of suspected disease with the maximum amount of radiation. Dr. David Gastineau, the head radiologist, was encouraging when he told me, "I think you were so doggone early in finding this and your health is so great and your blood tests are so good, that I just don't feel that the disease is elsewhere—I think we've cured you." Naturally that was good to hear. Nonetheless, I started to read everything I could about Hodgkin's disease. Although my Ph.D. is in business, I do have a master's degree in clinical psychology and a bachelor's degree in biology and chemistry, so that I have learned enough about science to be able to read and understand medical journals.

I read about Dr. Vera Peters, a prominent radiotherapist in Canada who specialized in Hodgkin's disease. There was evidence in one of her articles that if Hodgkin's disease was to be treated by radiation, it was best to treat the entire lymphatic system that might be involved, using a diagrammatic scheme that radiotherapists call the full Y. That means that they treat both sides of the neck, under both armpits, and down the middle of the chest to the upper abdomen—thereby they radiate all of the lymph nodes in those areas. If the Hodgkin's is confined to those areas, which it often is, it is curable. So I went back with this information to Dr. Gastineau and said, "I think it would pay if we were to treat the other side, under the right arm and do the right side of the neck," and he concurred. This was done as a prophylactic measure, a kind of insurance policy, even though it was kind of experimental at that time. This was in the middle of 1967 and I thought, well, maybe I am cured, but let's try to make sure. Perhaps it was sort of an overkill with radiation, but it was my prodding that caused Dr. Gastineau to agree to do the right side. He said, "Well, looking at Dr. Peters's reports, let's do it."

After the radiation I really thought I might be cured. Nonetheless, I was continuing my concerted effort to learn as much as I could about Hodgkin's disease to try to plan my strategy, in the event that I did relapse. Then in November 1968, about a year and a half later, I began running a little bit of a fever, and without any obvious signs of infection, that was an ominous sign. It meant that the Hodgkin's disease cancer cells, which often cause unexplained fever, could be anywhere in my body, and how would we ever get them all with additional radiation? So it didn't make sense to me to go back to radiation treatment. I had been hearing about the use of chemotherapy at Memorial Sloan-Kettering in New York and at the National Cancer Institute in Bethesda. The only thing that made sense to me was to go with some kind of chemical treatment that would circulate throughout my entire body and hopefully destroy those cells wherever they might be hiding.

I began to chart the course of my temperature. The fever was mild for about a month or so, but when it slowly began to increase, I went back to Dr. Gastineau. He decided to do a lymphangiogram, a procedure in which they put a kind of dye into the foot that flows through the lymphatic vessels to the lymph nodes of the pelvis and abdomen. Because the x-rays are blocked by the dye, it shows up on the x-ray picture and the radiologist can see if the lymph nodes are normal or distorted with tumors such as Hodgkin's disease. About that time my symptoms started to worsen: my fever was elevating and I had drenching sweats at night and severe itching, all of which are characteristic of recurrent Hodgkin's disease. Indeed the lymphangiogram showed disease in the lymph nodes deep in the abdomen, and with that information, my doctors recommended more radiation, but I refused. I wanted chemotherapy. I wanted the experimental treatment with a combination of four drugs, called the MOPP treatment, even though it was not fully approved. The procarbazine of the MOPP program wasn't approved by the FDA at that time, but I said that was the way I wanted to go and I had to go somewhere where they were willing to treat me. Dr. Gastineau said, "Fine, let me know what I can do," and he gave all kinds of support to my efforts.

I have a really good physician friend here in Fort Wayne who is a general practitioner. He wasn't a specialist in Hodgkin's disease, of course, but he said, "I'll go anywhere in the world with you, Les, that you want to go." And I asked him to come along because he would be able to open doors for me that I couldn't open because I'm not a physician. Another close friend of mine, Marvin E. Finn, was a pilot (so am I), and he offered to fly me wherever I wanted to go. So the three of us went to New York, and I went to Memorial Sloan-Kettering and asked to receive the MOPP treatment. I had taken along my x-rays and other medical records—Dr. Gastineau made sure I had everything along that the doctors would need—and my companion, Dr. Alan R. Chambers, was also available. At any rate, the doctors at Memorial said, "No, we're sorry, we won't give you the MOPP treatment. You've already had too much radiation and your body cannot stand the onslaught of the combination chemotherapy that is involved in the MOPP treatment. We just won't do it." I said, "Well, what's my choice—what do I do?" I had a high fever by this time, consistently around 102 or 103 degrees, and they said that the only thing that would help me was to take more radiation, and that's what they recommended for me.

I left there and went to the National Cancer Institute and presented my case. Some key physicians who were associated with the research program told me the same thing that I was told in New York, "No, you've had too much radiation, which damages your bone marrow, and we may kill you if we give you the MOPP treatment." By now I was really in bad shape, with raging fevers, shivering, and I couldn't think too clearly. I was wearing an overcoat because I was chilled, though I was running a high fever, and I felt just horrible. I decided that, since I could not think too clearly anymore, I might have to yield, and I went back to Dr. Gastineau and he said, "Les, I feel that we should at least treat the abdominal (retroperitoneal) area with radiation." And I agreed. The radiation helped, the symptoms subsided, and I could think clearly again.

At that time I decided to go to Birmingham to talk with Dr. Howard Skipper about some of his research. I had read about him, so I called and he said, "Sure, I'd be glad to see you." He called me back a little later and said, "Maybe you misunderstood, I'm not a physician, I can't treat you, I'm a Ph.D." I said, "Great, so am I, and I'd like to come see you." Howard was an absolute gem. He gave us about two hours of his time (again my two friends came with me). Dr. Skipper cleared up in my mind a lot of the things that I didn't quite understand about the theoretical background of the MOPP chemotherapy treatment, such as what the symptoms of Hodgkin's disease mean, and at what point the disease advances to become terminal. I then asked, "Dr. Skipper, can you tell me of anybody in the whole world who's an outstanding researcher in this field, but enough of a clinician that he might be willing to treat me? I've had considerable radiation, even more radiation than when they refused to treat me with this program at New York or NCI." He said, "Well, I think you want to talk to a fellow in Houston, Texas, by the name of Emil Frei III, at M. D. Anderson Hospital." I said, "Great, can I use your name?" and he said, "Certainly." Although I had only just met Dr. Skipper, he was still kind enough to let me use his name. So I called Dr. Frei and said I had been talking to Dr. Skipper. Dr. Frei asked, "Oh, how is Howard?" and I said, "He's just fine," like we were old friends.

I had been keeping my illness secret from most of my family and my associates, so I wanted to meet Dr. Frei on a weekend. He was kind enough to meet me on a Saturday morning in the clinic. Again I was loaded down with my x-rays and record, which he studied, and then he examined me. I brought along my blood counts, my temperature records, and a lot of other data as well. He went through all of this and at the end he said, "I think you're strong enough for the MOPP treatment, and I'll be willing to treat you." I said, "Say that to me again, I can't believe my ears!" He answered, "When do you want to start?" and I said, "How about now?" He started me out on the treatment, and then he sent Dr. Gastineau a sufficient amount of the drugs with instructions on how to give them. I personally carried some of that information, dealing with the precise dosages and so forth to give Dr. Gastineau so that he could follow the directions of Dr. Frei. I went through a series of MOPP (nitrogen mustard, oncovin or vincristine, procarbazine, and prednisone) treatments for six months.

The nitrogen mustard treatments, of course, raised Cain with me, but I took it in such a way that nobody knew I was taking it. Dr. Gastineau would administer the drug in the clinic on a Friday afternoon; then I would check into a motel room, because I knew I was going to be sicker than a dog for the weekend.

My wife knew what was going on, and so did my oldest child, but I didn't let my other four kids know. I purposely didn't want them to worry, in view of the fact that I was convinced somehow that I was going to cure myself. So why burden them at their early ages with a problem that may turn out not to be a problem? It's true I was ambivalent about what I ought to do with regard to the children. I had a very good friend who was a child psychologist and another good friend who was a child psychiatrist, and I got both of them together and laid it out for them. "Am I being selfish by not sharing such information with my kids, or am I proper in feeling I ought not to burden them with a very traumatic situation?" I thought I should ask these professionals to answer that question, rather than my trying to make the decision myself. What do you think happened? One of them said, "Tell the children," and the other said, "Don't tell the children." I laughingly chided them for not solving my dilemma, and I decided not to tell them. So I would check into the motel and become very very ill with nausea, vomiting, and diarrhea, and this would go on for hours. [Today, with the availability of potent antinausea and antivomiting medications, such serious gastrointestinal effects are quite uncommon.] But by the middle of the next day, around noon on Saturday, I felt halfway decent and could go back home, and no one was the wiser. By Monday morning I felt just fine and was back in my office working, and my colleagues didn't know about my illness. When you really look at it, it wasn't that bad. It was a matter of maybe fifteen hours that I was really sick, and within twenty-four hours I felt pretty human again. That was a small price to pay for life.

I kept up this routine for the six months Dr. Frei had intended as the duration of the treatment program. However, at my own insistence, because of what I had read, I felt I ought to go on a further program of maintenance chemotherapy. I kind of pressed Tom Frei on this. He said, "Well, there's not really good clean evidence that the maintenance chemotherapy is the way to go." And I said, "But is it going to hurt me?" And he said, "Well, probably not, but I really can't advise you to do it." And I said, "Well, will you do it if I insist?" and he said, "Yes." So we went that route, and I received the vinblastine (Velban) drug and kept that up for another year and a half. I believe I took it every two weeks by injection. That was kind of my insurance policy, and now the evidence is quite clear that it doesn't help in that circumstance, but we didn't know that at the time. It was my insisting that prompted Dr. Frei to give me the drug.

Fortunately, despite the considerable amount of radiation therapy that I had had, I was able to tolerate the other effects of chemotherapy quite well, and I have stayed well ever since. There has been no recurrence of my disease in a great many years. The last drug I took was the Velban back in 1971. I'd go back to see Tom Frei every six months or so, and I guess it must have been around 1975 before he said, "Well, it looks—" he never really would come right out and say, "Hey, don't sweat it, you're totally cured, forget it." He was being very very encouraging at four and five years, and then finally he said, "Let's extend your visits and make them every year instead of every six months." I keep going back, even now I go back yearly, not because I don't feel that the treatment has been successful, but because I happen to like the guy. We go out and have dinner and talk and enjoy each other's company. We have a lot in common. He's the same age I am, he's tall like I am, and we're both Catholics, we both have five kids, we're both ex-naval officers.

Without good researchers like Dr. Frei and Dr. Skipper and others, we certainly wouldn't be at the point we are today with respect to cures for cancer. Unless that pioneering work had been done with children with acute leukemia, they wouldn't have been able to cure people like me with Hodgkin's disease or other people with certain types of widespread cancer. I think there's a long way to go yet with research, and we need to invest much more money, both through government research programs and through other agencies like the American Cancer Society. We could save so many more lives with additional medical research in diseases like cancer and AIDS and others. We need to be very generous with our support of research, and I also think that there should be a huge carrot of a reward for the research specialist or individuals who come up with important medical cures.

Epilogue

A Disease
with Hope

Although we continue to learn a great deal about childhood acute lymphocytic leukemia, including how to cure it, we still do not know its causes. The disease increases in incidence about 1 percent per year, with far fewer dying of it because of improvements in therapy. Several large epidemiologic studies will be completed in the next few years that will tell us about such possible risk factors as living near electromagnetic power lines, occupational exposures of parents, and hazards of drugs. On the one hand, we do not presently believe that living near power lines or using cellular phones is important. On the other hand, the maternal use of alcohol or illicit drugs like marijuana, exposure to pesticides or radiation during pregnancy, and the father's preconception exposure to radiation (for example, diagnostic x-rays to the abdomen/spine, working with radiation) all confer added risk to the child for developing leukemia. Curiously, previous fetal loss by the mother greatly increases the risk. Another interesting report is that a child's frequent eating of hot dogs appears to increase the chances for developing leukemia. The underlying factor is presumably the use of nitrites, which can subsequently be metabolized into carcinogenic nitrosamines, in meat preservation. This remains to be confirmed, however.

It has been learned that many subtle variants of childhood acute lymphocytic leukemia occur, depending on which genes are abnormal. About half of all cases have translocated or improperly positioned chromosomes causing the leukemia, while in the rest there are mutations and deletions of critical genes. Whether the leukemic cell originates as a T- or B-cell type is important; T cells have a worse prognosis. The most favorable prognostic groups are B-cell leukemias in children under age ten who have no central nervous system involvement, a white blood cell count under 50,000 cells at the time of diagnosis, and an increase in DNA content of the leukemic cells. Such patients have about a 90 percent long-term survival rate. The cases with the poorest prognosis have about a 50 percent long-term survival rate.

Even with all our advances, the treatment of childhood leukemia requires special training and expertise. Today, fortunately, most major medical centers and children's hospitals have the capability to care for children with leukemia. There is still a fine line between what is called research and what is considered normal or accepted medical practice, and in my view, it is imperative to consult a specialist before treatment for a complex illness like leukemia is initiated. There are two major reasons for this. The first is that certain subtle clinical and laboratory features of each patient predict the likelihood of response to what may now be regarded as standard treatment. Thus a patient who has a more dangerous variety of leukemia, a so-called poor-risk patient, should be treated with a program that is different from that of the "average" patient. Careful individual tailoring of treatment is now yielding cures tending toward the 90 percent figure, although that remains to be confirmed. A 1994 study of four types of intensive treatment showed 95 percent disease-free survival at four years after remission.

Second, the only way to continue to ascend to the next level of success in understanding the disease and its treatments is to have each patient considered for enrollment in a clinical research study. Such a study involves the use of a specific protocol targeted to achieve more cures and/or to cause fewer side effects; successful conduct of such studies is where the next generation of advances must originate. We do know that patients who seem to be cured of leukemia are more susceptible to getting a second malignancy than is the average person, and this issue will require more study. Treatment with cytotoxic drugs increases the frequency of mutations that may lead to malignancies later in life. We are learning that some drugs are more dangerous in this respect, and they are being eliminated and replaced with safer drugs. Additionally, there are inherited factors that predispose one not only to one form of cancer or leukemia but also to others. For example, suppressor genes, a class of genes that function to prevent abnormally rapid cell growth, can be inactive in some children, greatly increasing their likelihood of developing multiple cancers. Fortunately this condition, which is known as the Li-Fraumeni Syndrome, is rare, but the principle could be important to others with cancer. The problem of sorting out later cancers that are due to the use of potent drugs from those caused by genetic susceptibility, or a combination thereof, is currently a very difficult matter.

The Children's Cancer Study Group, an important national study group headquartered in Arcadia, California, chaired by Dr. Denman Hammond, and involving many cooperating hospitals, has followed 2,400 patients for seven years or more after leukemia remission: second cancers were found in forty-four (1.8 percent) individuals. Other smaller studies suggest that the proportion may be higher, especially over a long lifetime. Thus there is still a concern that "cured" leukemia patients are at increased risk for cancer and other complications. We also know that of long-term survivors at St. Jude, about 80 percent have had no later health problems related to leukemia or its treatment, and this is a most important statistic.

Bone marrow transplantation is often the life-saving treatment of choice for a patient with a high-risk leukemia or a relapse, particularly in leukemia in adults. This is another highly technical, specialized, and expensive procedure. It may be combined with immune treatments, specially designed toxic antibodies to eliminate the remaining leukemic cells.

Exciting new biological treatments have evolved using growth factors that stimulate healthy bone marrow cells to recover while leukemia cells are being killed. Potent monoclonal antibodies are used to destroy the last remaining leukemic cells in a bone marrow sample removed from a high-risk patient during a remission. Such "cleansed" bone marrow is then available to reinfuse, should that become necessary. Recent developments in the area of biological growth factors have provided a potentially unlimited supply of factors to stimulate the growth of normal white blood cells, red blood cells—and soon we will have it for platelets as well. This technology promises to revolutionize the management of acute leukemia. Further improvements in bone marrow transplantation are expected to greatly increase the compatibility of donors—enabling more patients to receive life-saving treatment.

Gene therapy is something else that is rapidly changing from fantasy to possibility to reality. The ability to use "anti-sense" molecules to switch off the abnormal genes that power leukemic cells, to insert suppressor genes that modulate or tame malignant growth, and to cause normal bone marrow cells to become resistant to chemotherapy drugs (thereby enabling

269

the use of higher doses of leukemia-killing drugs) are all remarkable approaches being pioneered at this time.

Then there are revolutionary new ideas emerging about how to induce leukemic cells to become "more normal" in their behavior, a prospect that might someday eliminate the need for toxic drugs altogether. For example, adult acute promyelocytic leukemia responds remarkably to treatment with a vitamin A–like substance called retinoic acid. First found to be a maturing factor in tissue culture of leukemic cells, it has led to a new kind of biological therapy that is far more effective even than chemotherapy for this type of leukemia.

In citing new possibilities in gene therapy and in using drugs to induce leukemic cells to behave more like normal cells, it is appropriate to tie these together with a most exciting new area called programmed cell death, or apoptosis. In a review article on the subject, Leo Sacks and J. Lotem describe the process by which normal adult cells, such as those in the skin, bowel, or blood, come to the end of their life span and are replaced by new cells. Disruption of this normal process of cell death can give rise to certain types of leukemia and cancer by causing such cells to appear to be immortal. Unexpectedly, however, cytotoxic chemotherapy and drugs like retinoids, or the replacement of faulty suppressor genes, like p53 or bcl-2, can restore programmed cell death. Is restoration of normal apoptosis the common element of a lasting remission, regardless of how it is achieved? Currently these are potential new avenues for treatment; with additional research, one can hope that they will become realities soon.

The most frustrating aspect of using chemotherapy to treat malignancies like leukemia is that, unless the malignant cells are destroyed, they eventually become resistant to the drugs used to cause the initial improvement. We have learned that leukemic cell resistance takes many forms. A drug like vincristine can be pumped out of a resistant cell as though the cell has a special vacuum cleaner. Other drugs like methotrexate can be blocked from entering a resistant cell in the first place, fail to be metabolized to their most active form, or come up against a cell that has synthesized more of the target enzyme (dihydrofolate reductose) than can possibly be inhibited by the drugs. These are some of the many ways that the leukemia cell can overcome our drugs. But uncovering these mechanisms of drug resistance has also provided many new avenues to circumvent the problems.

Perhaps by understanding how and when the crucial leukemia-causing mutations occur we will eventually learn to prevent the disease altogether—which would be the greatest blessing of all. But that discovery will probably take a decade or longer to achieve. Clearly there is no shortage of creative ideas, only of money to support the work. We must redouble our efforts to keep the conquest of leukemia on track by raising money to do the research that begs to be done and to attract the next generation of leaders into cancer and leukemia research. How high is cancer research among our priorities in this country? Repeated polls show it to be the top health priority for our citizens. Yet in the eyes of our government, and in terms of the level of donations to the not-for-profit organizations that support cancer research, it is not nearly high enough a priority to fuel the progress that could be made by scientists here and now. The truism prevails in these endeavors that the budget *is* the message.

While we are learning about the genetic changes that are responsible for the development of leukemia in the first place, striking practical applications of current knowledge are still ahead. It is remarkable how much more basic information is now available than was known to the pioneers in leukemia research. And there is no doubt that Burchenal, Frei, Freireich, and all of the others are right—as further advances are made in leukemia they will add new and critical pieces of information toward the cure of other, more common cancers. Thanks to these productive researchers and their many colleagues, medical science has been changed for all time. Still there exists ample room, and many challenging opportunities, for the next generation of pioneers who are even now pondering their choice of career. It will not be nearly as difficult to make the next set of advances as it was to make the first ones.

It is my belief that we are on the threshold of real progress in managing cancer. Leukemia research has played a major role in understanding the larger principles of treatment. Whole new horizons are appearing as we learn to combine these principles with the more fundamental understandings of cancer growth and development. I make no rash promises or predictions. But if the past is prologue, then the story of cancer will eventually have a happy ending. In the meantime, none of our researchers will rest until all forms of leukemia are completely curable.

Bibliography

History of Leukemia

Bender, George A. *Great Moments in Medicine*. Detroit: Parke-Davis, 1961. Published by a pharmaceutical company, this excellent and very readable book describes some of the great people and discoveries in medicine.

Biermer, D. "Ein Fall von Leukaemie." *Virchows Archives* 20 (1861): 552–554. Original case description of leukemia in a child—the basis of the chapter on Maria.

Burchenal, J. H. "From Wild Fowl to Stalking Horses: Alchemy in Chemotherapy." Fifth Annual David A. Karnofsky Memorial Lecture. *Cancer* 35, no. 4 (1975): 1121–1135. History of chemotherapy from ancient times and the importance of chemotherapy in leukemia treatment. From a lecture honoring a former friend and colleague of Dr. Burchenal.

———. "The Historical Development of Cancer Chemotherapy." *Seminars in Oncology* 6 (1979): 490–505. Chemotherapy has a venerable past, well reviewed in this article, but a rather technical approach that will appeal to people with a good chemistry background.

DeVita, V. T., Serpick, A. A., and Carbone, P. P. "Combination Chemotherapy in the Treatment of Advanced Hodgkin's Disease." *Annals of Internal Medicine* 73 (1970): 881–895. Key contribution in the cure of Hodgkin's disease.

Farber, S., Diamond, L. K., Mercer, R. D., et al. "Temporary Remissions in Acute Leukemia in Children Produced by Folic Acid Antagonist, 4-Aminopteroylglutamic Acid (Aminopterin)." *New England Journal of Medicine* 238 (1948): 787. First well-documented remissions in childhood leukemia with chemotherapy. This classic paper initiated the quest to cure leukemia.

Freireich, E. J, and Lemak, N. A. *Milestones in Leukemia Research and Therapy*. Baltimore and London: Johns Hopkins University Press, 1991. Splendid history and references for professionals; highly recommended for students of cancer research.

Bibliography

Goodman, L. S., Wintrobe, M. M., Dameshek, W., et al. "Use of Methyl-Bis(Beta-Chloroethyl)amine Hydrochloride and Tris(Beta-Chloroethyl)amine Hydrochloride for Hodgkin's Disease, Lymphosarcoma, Leukemia and Certain Allied and Miscellaneous Disorders." *Journal of the American Medical Association* 132 (1948): 126–132. Classic article on chemotherapy with alkylating agents for Hodgkin's disease and leukemia.

Gunz, F. W., and Henderson, E. S., eds. *Leukemia*. New York: Grune & Stratton, 1983. A clearly written text for students and doctors.

Haddow, A. "Thoughts on Chemical Therapy." David A. Karnofsky Memorial Lecture. *Cancer* 26 (1970): 737–754. By one of the most imaginative leaders in modern cancer chemotherapy.

Hayhoe, F.G.J. *Leukemia: Research and Clinical Practice*. Boston: Little, Brown, and Co. 1960. Nice historical account of the recognition of leukemia as a distinct disease.

Leuchtenberger, C., Leuchtenberger, R., Laszlo, D., et al. "Folic Acid, a Tumor Growth Inhibitor." *Proceedings of the Society for Experimental Biology and Medicine* 55 (1944): 204. On the importance of nutritional factors for the growth of cancer cells in mice, an important step that led to the development of folate antagonists.

Li, M. C., Hertz, R., and Spencer, D. B. "Effect of Methotrexate upon Choriocarcinoma and Chorioadenoma." *Proceedings of the Society for Experimental Biology and Medicine* 93 (1956): 361–366. Important progress in the treatment of a widespread cancer, which later would be the first to be cured by chemotherapy alone. Many lessons from the treatment of this rare cancer were applied to leukemia.

Pochedly, L. "Dr. James A. Wolff II: First Successful Chemotherapy of Acute Leukemia." *American Journal of Pediatric Hematology/Oncology* 6 (1984): 449–453. Personal reminiscences of work in Boston with Dr. Sidney Farber.

Rolleston, H. "The History of Haematology." *Proceedings of the Royal Society of Medicine* 27 (1934): 1161–1178. Scholarly, beautifully written early history of investigations of leukemia, blood cells.

Sturgis, C. C. *Hematology*, 2d ed. Springfield, Ill.: Charles C. Thomas, 1955. Chapter 16. Scholarly review of the early leukemia literature.

Tucker, Jonathan B. *Ellie: A Child's Fight against Leukemia*. New York: Holt, Rinehart and Winston, 1982. A touching, personal story of a child's bravery in the fight against leukemia. Many of the medical experiences are clearly explained in lay terminology.

Virchow, R. *Gesammelte Abhandlugen zur Wissenschaftlichem Medicine*. Frankfurt: Merdinger Sohn & Co., 1856. First pathology description of leukemia by the pathologist who discovered the cellular nature of cancer and leukemia.

Zubrod, C. G. "Historic Milestones in Curative Chemotherapy." *Seminars in Oncology* 6 (1979): 490–505. Perspective of one of the most highly regarded leaders in the search for a cure.

Other Important Articles and Reviews

Acute Leukemia Group B. "New Treatment Schedule with Improved Survival in Childhood Leukemia." *Journal of the American Medical Association* 194, no. 1 (1965): 75–81.

Aur, R.J.A., Simone, J., Hustu, H. O., Walters, T., Borella, L., Pratt, C., and Pinkel, D. "Central Nervous System Therapy and Combination Chemotherapy of Childhood Lymphocytic Leukemia." *Blood* 37, no. 3 (1971): 272–281.

Burchenal, J. H. "History of Intrathecal Prophylaxis and Therapy of Meningeal Leukemia." *Cancer Drug Delivery* 1 (1983): 87–92.

Burchenal, J. H., Ellison, R. R., Murphy, M. C., et al. "Clinical Studies on 6-Mercaptopurine." *Annals of the New York Academy of Sciences* 60 (1954): 359–368.

Burchenal, J. H., and Murphy, M. C. "Long-term Survivors in Acute Leukemia." *Cancer Research* 25 (1965): 1491–1494.

Clarke, D. A., Elion, G. B., Hitchings, G. H., and Stock, C. C. "Structure-Activity Relationships among Purines Related to 6-Mercaptopurine." *Cancer Research* 18, no. 4 (1958): 445–456.

Elion, G. B. "Biochemistry and Pharmacology of Purine Analogues." *Federation Proceedings* 26, no. 3 (1967): 898–904.

Elion, G. B., Callahan, S. W., Hitchings, G. H., Rundles, R. W., and Laszlo, J. "Experimental Clinical and Metabolic Studies of Thiopurines." *Cancer Chemotherapy Reports*, no. 16 (1962): 197–202.

Elion, G. B., Callahan, S., Rundles, R. W., and Hitchings, G. H. "Relationship between Metabolic Fates and Antitumor Activities of Thiopurines." *Cancer Research* 23, no. 8 (1963): 1207–1217.

Elion, G. B., Hitchings, G. H., and Vanderwerff, H. "Antagonists of Nucleic Acid Derivatives." *Journal of Biological Chemistry* 192, no. 2 (1951): 505–518.

Ellison, R. R., Holland, J. F., Weil, M., Jacquillat, C., Boiron, M., et al. "Arabinosyl Cytosine: A Useful Agent in the Treatment of Acute Leukemia in Adults." *Blood* 32, no. 4 (1968): 507–523.

Freeman, A. I., . . . Holland, J. F. "Comparison of Intermediate-dose Methotrexate with Cranial Irradiation for the Post-Induction Treatment of Acute Lymphocytic Leukemia in Children." *New England Journal of Medicine* 308 (1983): 477–484.

Frei, E., III. "Combination Cancer therapy: Presidential Address." *Cancer Research* 32, no. 12 (1972): 2593–2607.

———. "Selected Considerations Regarding Chemotherapy as Adjuvant in Cancer Treatment." *Cancer Chemotherapy Reports* 50 (1966): 1–8.

Frei, E., III, DeVita, V. T., Moxley, J. H., III, and Carbone, P. P. "Approaches to Improving the Chemotherapy of Hodgkin's Disease." *Cancer Research* 26, pt. 1 (1966): 1284–1289.

Frei, E., III, and Freireich, E. J. "Progress and Perspectives in the Chemotherapy of Acute Leukemia." *Advances in Chemotherapy* 2 (1965): 269–298.

Frei, E., III, Freireich, E. J, Gehan, E., Pinkel, D., Holland, J. F., et al. "Studies of

Sequential and Combination Antimetabolite Therapy in Acute Leukemia: 6-Mercaptopurine and Methotrexate." *Blood* 18, no. 4 (1961): 431–453.

Frei, E., III, Holland, J. F., Schneiderman, M. A., Pinkel, D., Selkirk, G., Freireich, E. J, Silver, R. T., Gold, G. L., and Regelson, W. "A Comparative Study of Two Regimes of Combination Chemotherapy in Acute Leukemia." *Blood* 13, no. 12 (1958): 1126–1148.

Frei, E., III, Karon, M., Levin, R. H., Freireich, E. J, et al. "The Effectiveness of Combinations of Antileukemic Agents in Inducing and Maintaining Remission in Children with Acute Leukemia." *Blood* 26, no. 5 (1965): 642–656.

Frei, E., III, Rosowsky, A., Wright, J. E., Cucchi, C. A., Lippke, J. A., Ervin, T. J., Jolivet, J., and Haseltine, W. A. "Development of Methotrexate Resistance in a Human Squamous Cell Carcinoma of the Head and Neck in Culture." *Proceedings of the National Academy of Sciences USA* 81 (1984): 2873–2877.

Freireich, E. J, and Frei, E., III. "Recent Advances in Acute Leukemia." *Progress in Hematology* 4 (1964): 187–202.

Freireich, E. J, Frei, E., III, Holland, J. F., Pinkel, D., Selawry, O., Rothberg, H., Haurani, F., Taylor, R., and Gehan, E. A. "Evaluation of a New Chemotherapeutic Agent in Patients with 'Advanced Refractory' Acute Leukemia: Studies of 6-Azauracil." *Blood* 16, no. 3 (1960): 1268–1278.

Freireich, E. J, Gehan, E., Frei, E., III, Schroeder, L. R., Wolman, R. A., Burgert, E. O., Mills, S. D., Pinkel, D., Selawry, O. S., Moon, J. H., Gendel, B. R., Spurr, C. L., Storrs, R., Haurani, F., Hoogstraten, B., and Lee, S. "The Effect of 6-Mercaptopurine on the Duration of Steroid-induced Remissions in Acute Leukemia: A Model for Evaluation of Other Potentially Useful Therapy." *Blood* 21, no. 6 (1963): 699–716.

Freireich, E. J, Gehan, E. A., Rall, D. P., Schmidt, L. H., and Skipper, H. E. "Quantitative Comparison of Toxicity of Anticancer Agents in Mouse, Rat, Hamster, Dog, Monkey, and Man." *Cancer Chemotherapy Reports* 50 (1966): 219–244.

Freireich, E. J, Gehan, E. A., Sulman, D., Boggs, D. R., and Frei, E., III. "The Effect of Chemotherapy on Acute Leukemia in the Human." *Journal of Chronic Diseases* 14, no. 6 (1961): 593–608.

Freireich, E. J, Henderson, E. S., Karon, M. R., and Frei, E., III. "The Treatment of Acute Leukemia Considered with Respect to Cell Population Kinetics." *The Proliferation and Spread of Neoplastic Cells: 21st Annual Symposium on Fundamental Cancer Research* (1967): 441–452.

Freireich, E. J, Judson, G., and Levin, R. H. "Separation and Collection of Leukocytes." *Cancer Research* 25 (1965): 1516–1520.

Freireich, E. J, Kliman, A., Gaydos, L. A., Mantel, N., and Frei, E., III. "Response to Repeated Platelet Transfusion from the Same Donor." *Annals of Internal Medicine* 59, no. 3 (1963): 277–287.

Freireich, E. J, Levin, R. H., Whang, J., Carbone, P. O., Bronson, W., and Morse, E. E. "The Function and Fate of Transfused Leukocytes from Donors with Chronic Myelocytic Leukemia in Leukopenic Recipients." *Annals of the New York Academy of Sciences* 113, art. 2 (1964): 1081–1089.

Freireich, E. J, Schmidt, P. J., Schneiderman, M. A., et al. "A Comparative Study of the Effect of Transfusion of Fresh and Preserved Whole Blood on Bleeding in Patients with Acute Leukemia." *New England Journal of Medicine* 260 (1959): 6–11.

George, P., Hernandex, K., Hustu, O., Borella, L., Holton, C., and Pinkel, D. "A Study of 'Total Therapy' of Acute Lymphocytic Leukemia in Children." *Journal of Pediatrics* 72, no. 3 (1968): 399–408.

Hitchings, G. H. "The Bertner Foundation Memorial Award Lecture: Salmon, Butterflies, and Cancer Chemotherapy," pp. 25–43. In *Symposium on Fundamental Cancer Research, 1974: Pharmacological Basis of Cancer Chemotherapy.* Baltimore: Williams & Wilkins Co., 1975.

Hitchings, G. H. "Chemotherapy and Comparative Biochemistry." G.H.A. Clowes Memorial Lecture. *Cancer Research* 29 (1969): 1895–1903.

Hitchings, G. H. "A Quarter Century of Chemotherapy." *Journal of the American Medical Association* 209, no. 9 (1969): 1339–1340.

Hitchings, G. H., and Elion, G. B. "The Chemistry and Biochemistry of Purine Analogs." *Annals of the New York Academy of Sciences* 60 (1954): 195–199.

———. "Mechanisms of Action of Purine and Pyrimidine Analogues," pp. 26–36. In *Cancer Chemotherapy*, ed. I. Brodsky and S. B. Kahn. New York: Grune & Stratton, 1967.

———. "Purine and Pyrimidine Analogs in Cancer Chemotherapy." *GANN Monograph No. 6* (1968): 5–13.

Holland, J. F. "Clinical Studies of Unmaintained Remissions in Acute Lymphocytic Leukemia." *The Proliferation and Spread of Neoplastic Cells: 21st Annual Symposium on Fundamental Cancer Research* (1967): 453–462.

———. "Combination Therapy of Acute Lymphocytic Leukemia of Children." *Journal of the American Medical Association* 222, no. 9 (1972): 1169–1170.

———. "E Pluribus Unum: Presidential Address." *Cancer Research* 31 (1971): 1319–1329.

———. "Intensive High Dose Treatment of Children in Complete Remission of Acute Lymphocytic Leukemia," pp. 163–169. In *Treatment of Burkitt's Tumour*, ed. J. H. Burchenal and D. P. Burkitt. UICC Monograph Series, vol. 8. 1967.

———. "Who Should Treat Acute Leukemia?" *Journal of the American Medical Association* 209, no. 10 (1969): 1511–1513.

Jaffe, N., Frei, E., III, Traggis, D., and Bishop, Y. "Adjuvant Methotrexate and Citrovorum-factor Treatment of Osteogenic Sarcoma." *New England Journal of Medicine* 29, no. 19 (1974): 994–997.

Leventhal, B. G., Levine, A. S., Graw, R. G., Jr., Simon, R., Freireich, E. J, and Henderson, E. S. "Long-term Second Remissions in Acute Lymphatic Leukemia." *Cancer* 35, no. 4 (1975): 1136–1140.

Pinkel, D. "Allogenic Bone Marrow Transplantation in Children with Acute Leukemia: A Practice Whose Time Has Gone." *Leukemia* 3 (1988): 242–244.

Bibliography

————. "Curing Children of Leukemia." *Cancer* 59, no. 10 (1987): 1683–1691.

————. "Five-Year Follow-up of 'Total Therapy' of Childhood Lymphocytic Leukemia." *Journal of the American Medical Association* 216, no. 4 (1971): 648–652.

Pinkel, D., Hernandex, K., Borella, L., Holton, C., Aur, R., Samoy, G., and Pratt, C. "Drug Dosage and Remission Duration in Childhood Lymphocytic Leukemia." *Cancer* 27, no. 2 (1971): 247–256.

Pinkel, D., Simone, J., Hustu, H. O., Aur, R.J.A. "Nine Years' Experience with 'Total Therapy' of Childhood Acute Lymphocytic Leukemia." *Pediatrics* 50, no. 2 (1972): 246–251.

Rai, K. R., Holland, J. F., Glidewell, O. J., et al. "Treatment of Acute Myelocytic Leukemia: A Study by Cancer and Leukemia Group B." *Blood* 58, no. 6 (1981): 1203–1212.

Rivera, G. K., Pinkel, D., Simone, J. W., et al. "Treatment of Acute Lymphoblastic Leukemia." *New England Journal of Medicine* 329 (1993): 1289–1295.

Sacks, L., and Lotem, J. "Control of Programmed Cell Death in Normal and Leukemic Cells: New Implications of Therapy" *Blood* 82 (1993): 15–21.

Skipper, H. E. "Dose Intensity versus Total Dose of Chemotherapy: An Experimental Basis," pp. 43–64. In *Important Advances in Oncology, 1990,* (ed. V. T. DeVita, Jr., S. Hellman, and S. A. Rosenberg). Philadelphia: J. B. Lippincott Co., 1990.

Skipper, H. E., and Bennett, L. L., Jr. "Biochemistry of Cancer." *Annual Review of Biochemistry* 27 (1958): 137–166.

Skipper, H. E., Heidelberger, C., and Welch, A. D. "Some Biochemical Problems of Cancer Chemotherapy." *Nature* 179 (1957): 1159–1162.

Skipper, H. E., Schabel, F. M., Jr., and Wilcox, W. S. "Experimental Evaluation of Potential Anticancer Agents. XIII. On the Criteria and Kinetics Associated with 'Curability' of Experimental Leukemias." *Cancer Chemotherapy* 35 (1964): 1–111.

Steinberg, P. G., Redner, A., Steinberg, L., et al. "Development of a New Intensive Therapy for Acute Lymphoblastic Leukemia in Children at Increased Risk of Early Relapse." *Cancer* 72 (1993): 3120–3130.

Yates, J., Glidewell, O., Wiernik, P., . . . (Holland, J. F.), et al. "Cytosine Arabinoside with Daunorubicin or Adriamycin for Therapy of Acute Myelocytic Leukemia: A CALGB Study." *Blood* 60, no. 2 (1982): 454–462.

Index

About the Author

Dr. John Laszlo, the National Vice President for Research of the American Cancer Society, brings a lifetime of medical experience—as physician, scientist, and cancer survivor—to this engrossing account of the cure of childhood leukemia. Dr. Laszlo's medical research interest began as a child, helping his father, Dr. Daniel Laszlo, test therapeutic substances from yeast and barley on tumors in mice. After taking his bachelor's degree at Columbia University in 1952 and his M.D. degree at Harvard University in 1955, he did both fundamental and clinical research on the behavior of leukemic blood cells and on the development of anticancer drugs at the National Cancer Institute and then at Duke University Medical School. He volunteered for the first test of a new blood cell separator and used the new technology to save the life of a desperately ill leukemia patient—experiences he recounts in this book. At the American Cancer Society (a not-for-profit agency), he oversees the largest nongovernmental cancer research program in the world. Dr. Laszlo has collaborated on leukemia research with many of the scientists and physicians whose stories he tells in *The Cure of Childhood Leukemia: Into the Age of Miracles*. He is the author of *Antiemetics and Cancer Chemotherapy* (Williams & Wilkins, 1983), a book for clinicians, and *Understanding Cancer* (Harper & Row, 1987), a book for the general public, as well as over two hundred scientific publications related to cancer and leukemia.